Under the Rainbow Moon

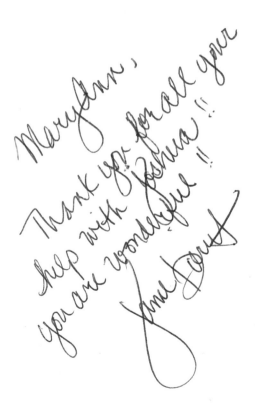

Under the Rainbow Moon

Hope and Healing for Lyme

JAMIE BIERUT

TATE PUBLISHING
AND ENTERPRISES, LLC

Published by Tate Publishing & Enterprises, LLC
127 E. Trade Center Terrace | Mustang, Oklahoma 73064 USA
1.888.361.9473 | www.tatepublishing.com

Tate Publishing is committed to excellence in the publishing industry. The company reflects the philosophy established by the founders, based on Psalm 68:11,
"The Lord gave the word and great was the company of those who published it."

Book design copyright © 2012 by Tate Publishing, LLC. All rights reserved.

Cover design inspired from artwork by Christi Ziebarth
Cover design by Rtor Maghuyop
Interior design by Jake Muelle

Published in the United States of America

ISBN: 978-1-62147-240-7
1. Medical, Healing
2. Biography & Autobiography, Personal Memoirs
12.08.15

DEDICATION

Dave, my soul mate, fifteen years ago we committed our lives together. Although we never anticipated this journey, we have embraced it with unity. Joshua could not have been given a more devoted and loyal father. I love you sweetly, honor you fervently, and cherish you forever. Your support, patience, and encouragement throughout the writing process are treasured. I want to continue to grow old with you and nurture an intimacy that knows no fear. Together we will fill our home with laughter and gentleness in Christ's love.

Alexa, you will always be my darling little girl even though you are turning into a beautiful young woman before my very eyes. My beautiful, nature loving, soccer player—I can't imagine life without you. You are my inspiration as well as your brother's protector, entertainer, and big sister. Loving Joshua will impact your life forever and bring glory to God's name.

Joshua, my sweet son, can you fathom how much you are loved? Never forget that you are beautifully and wonderfully made. You light up my life.

Caleb, Boo, you are a gift. You are my constant reminder that God knows my deepest needs. I see behind your huge, sparkly, blue eyes the wonder of life and the blessings of raising sons. My little chatterbox you will always be. So gregarious and full of life, you teach your brother what joy means.

ACKNOWLEDGEMENTS

It is my most humble privilege to remember and express my deepest thank so many who have turned my dreams of publishing a manuscript into reality.

My mothers (Mom and the "Other Mom"), you are my biggest cheerleaders. Your kind words and encouragement reminds me that I am worthy of love. Without your counsel, I really don't know if I would have had the strength to navigate the tenuous role of motherhood. The lengths that each of you have gone to for Joshua are astounding. I love you both so much.

Christi, you are my forever September 26, 1972, unconscious, penicillin, sulfa, IC, not-to-be-temptified, ever-flapping, trying-to-soar, best friend. Without you, I have no story to tell. Your wisdom, insight, words, and prayers have inspired me to keep running the race. Our God-ordained friendship valiantly withstands the test of time and proximity. Our cord of three strands will not easily be broken!

Janis McLaughlin, my dearest friend in Plymouth who has listened endlessly, comforted, and encouraged me throughout the entire writing process. You were always there for me the next morning with a cup of coffee and a smile after an endless night of writing.

Pastor Stan, you have filled the role of friend and father and have always known what I needed before I could even recognize it. Thank you for always believing in me and discipling me.

Plymouth United Methodist Church has always prayed for our family and surrounded us with love during the tough times.

Dr. Jones, nothing happens by accident. Our paths have crossed and life is enriched because of your mercy and kindness.

Words cannot express the gratitude and respect I have for you and your mission to help children with Lyme disease. I have never met a physician with more compassion or tenderness; you truly are an angel. Thank you for healing my son. Joshua is truly one of your pearls!

Dr. Stromberg, our pediatric psychiatrist who had the insight and creativity to think outside of the box and test for Lyme disease, changing our lives forever.

Dr. Mahan, who has given my son his happy feet and a better quality of life, free from foot pain.

Mary Ann McDonnell, Joshua's psychiatrist, to whom I am indebted for her availability and expertise in the world of bipolar disorder.

Tate Publishing, who believed in me, invested in me, and brought me to a higher level of writing I never dreamt possible.

All those that I have met and worked with have continuously urged me to write a book so that I could share my insight and faith, heal my broken heart, and make a difference in this world.

And last, but not least, God, who has guided, nurtured, and led me down this path with Joshua, and through the writing process to bring glory to His name.

TABLE OF CONTENTS

Part 1

Part 2

Part 3

PREFACE

"For I know the plans I have for you," declares the LORD,
"plans to prosper you and not to harm you, plans to give
you hope and a future."

Jeremiah 29:11

This verse resonated in my heart and mind when my second
child, Joshua David Bierut, entered into this world. He
was loved by me and my husband Dave before he was even born.
He was loved by the Lord before he ever was.

> You made all the delicate, inner parts of my body and
> knit me together in my mother's womb. Thank you for
> making me so wonderfully complex! Your workmanship
> is marvelous—how well I know it. You watched me as
> I was being formed in utter seclusion, as I was woven
> together in the dark of the womb. You saw me before
> I was born. Every day of my life was recorded in your
> book. Every moment was laid out before a single day had
> passed.

Psalm139: 13-16 (NLT)

My journey through both the beauty and wilderness of
parenting this child with special needs continues strong for
nearly twelve years, yet the extreme highs and lows of this
adventure make it seem like a lifetime. I have lived and breathed
a mother's fierce love. I have carried a fiery passion for my son.
I have owned many fears on wakeful nights and discovered
glimmers of hope by day. It's no wonder that I barely remember
my life without him in my world. This is our story.

I pray that I can articulate with precision and grace the depth and height of the pain and joy that transpires when you are blessed with a child with special needs. I pray there is at least one person out in this great big world that makes a connection with this journey, realizing they are never alone.

I have been given a passion and ability for writing, but I never have written for God's glory until now. Tonight I find myself being still amidst the chaos in my life. I feel God tugging on my sleeve and whispering in my ear to share our story with others. He's nudging me to make sense of the hope, grief, love, fear, and passion that lives inside every parent with whom God entrusts a child with special needs to raise.

PART 1

NEW BEGINNINGS

When my prince charming married me, it was a beautiful spring day—April 12, 1997. The tulips and daffodils were in bloom, and the sunbeams shone down, covering us with God's grace. We were young, in love, and believed that together we could conquer the world. Part of what made our relationship strong was our shared dreams; we wanted to begin a legacy filled with family and faith. Dave and I were eager to start a family and find common ground for our spiritual beliefs.

Dave's childhood was spent in New England where his family was very active in the Catholic Church. However, as adolescence approached, the family's involvement decreased. Conversely, I was raised in the Midwest at a Protestant Church. My mother took me and my sister Jessica to Sunday school every week. Although I was taught about a good man named Jesus, there was no personal relationship with Him.

With such divergent backgrounds, Dave and I were struggling to find the right religion for ourselves. Wanting to find common spiritual ground, we started attending Blackhawk Baptist Church in Fort Wayne, Indiana. Blackhawk was an independent Baptist Church which allowed us to become involved in its worship ministry before we were true believers.

I will be forever thankful for Blackhawk's welcoming arms. They allowed us to join the praise choir which exposed us to fellow Christians walking in faith. It was the catalyst which changed our lives and made us into the people we are today. We were newlyweds in love, excited about our new church home. Even more exhilarating, I became pregnant five months after our wedding.

ALEXA BROOKLIN

Nine months later our baby girl, Alexa Brooklin was born. We were enamored with this precious life God helped us create. Now, more than ever, I saw the enormity of raising my child up in faith, but I didn't understand how. After listening to the Word for nearly a year, I scheduled an appointment with Pastor Russell.

On Friday, July 24, 1998, with my baby girl in my arms, I asked him many reflective questions about faith, life, good, evil, heaven, and hell. That was the day my life was transformed forever. In Pastor Russell's tiny little office, I drew a line in the sand and chose to believe in my heart that God sent his son Jesus to die for my sins. I acknowledged Jesus as my personal Savior! Two days later my husband also offered his life to Jesus. We now had a foundation and faith to cling to and an amazing journey to embark on for our young family.

The first two years of Alexa's life were pure joy. She was everything we could have dreamed of in a little girl. She was affectionate, inquisitive, sweet, and precocious. Ahead of every developmental milestone, she made parenting seem easy. When she was twelve months old, we attended a Christian parenting series that provided direction for our parenting skills. Brought up upon Christian principles and a desire to raise children to high moral standards, this seemed like the perfect method for us to educate, love, and discipline.

Life was good, and it was simple. I was complete, I felt happier than ever before. Since parenting Alexa was so beautiful and natural, we figured two of her would be even better!

I learned quickly that if I had pregnancy on my mind or if I looked or breathed in the proper direction, I could inevitably become pregnant at the blink of an eye. Within one month, we were pregnant again with our second child.

JOSHUA DAVID

During my second pregnancy, patience was definitely not my virtue as I yearned to meet this sweet, precious baby. Jessica nicknamed the baby "mommy's little soccer player" because there was relentless kicking and constant activity. I couldn't breathe and my lungs felt squashed, as if I were desperate for each breath during the last few months. I begged and pleaded with my obstetrician, Dr. Walters, to induce me early due to my pain and discomfort. She relented, and the baby was scheduled to be born on July 24, 2000.

Hindsight delivers insight that nothing regarding this baby's birth was typical. The morning of delivery, I was late for arrival. (I am never late!) Dave drove like Fred Flintstone taking Wilma to Parkview Hospital. *What if the entire procedure is delayed now?* I thought. Thankfully, the nurses did not turn me away; they quickly admitted me and got our family's party back on schedule.

Since this was my first inducement procedure, I was startled to have an initial mind- blowing contraction within six measly minutes after the Pitocin drip started. Startled and scared. Dave went down for breakfast just as the drip was starting. He left me smiling and chatting away with the nurses, only to return fifteen minutes later to see me clutching the bedrails for dear life. The Pitocin was instigating intense, piercing, fiery hot waves of pain every five minutes. Instantly the baby went into fetal distress as the heart rate and oxygen saturation levels plummeted. Uncertainty and distress cascaded over me like a tidal wave. *Save my baby! Dear Lord, is the cord wrapped around its neck?* I thought.

Thankfully I was blessed to be in the care of competent, compassionate nurses who knew exactly what to do. Within one minute they administered oxygen, flipped me on my left side, and broke my water. Next they inserted a fetal monitor into the baby's skull. A few minutes stretched into a lifetime until finally the baby's heart rate and oxygen level increased.

Although the inducement was too traumatic for the tiny baby to handle, my baby already possessed a relentless instinct and determination to greet the world. Our anticipation climaxed with the shouts of joy, "It's a *boy!*" We were thrilled. *Thank you, Jesus! Thank you, Jesus!* But this baby entered the world stunned. The silence permeated our senses while we waited, anticipating his first breath of life.

I asked if he had all his fingers and toes and everyone laughed, "Yes!" He finally cried out with a mighty wail—apparently he needed to make a dramatic entrance. *What if my baby is already making a statement? What if he will always have trouble acclimating to his new world?* This fleeting thought wafted in and then back out of my mind once I gazed into his yellow-hazel, doe eyes. I was smitten. Head over heels in love with his breath, so clean and pure, and his skin, so smooth and delicate. He was two years younger than his sister and perfect in every way.

His name was Joshua David. His first name, Joshua, was in respect to Joshua, the Old Testament Israeli leader. David was in honor of his father, as well as the mighty warrior king David. Combined, these names exuded strength and leadership for his future. Life continued smoothly and seamlessly, and I felt God's presence in our lives whenever I looked at my two beautiful children.

God, you've given me the perfect family! How could I be so lucky! I am humbled by your blessings! Everything is perfect! I thought.

GOD DANCED

While adapting to life with another child back at home, I received one of the most endearing gifts of my life from my dear friend Marie Harrer. My mother was staying the week to help with the baby. We had just sat down for one of her delicious home cooked meals. As we attempted to take our first bite, the doorbell unexpectedly rang. We were interrupted by a Federal Express Carrier who was at our doorstep delivering me a package, shouting, "Special delivery for the mother of Joshua Bierut!"

I devoured the package wrappings instead of my meal, and inside I found the most beautiful picture with blue matting inside an oak frame. In rainbow colors it said "Joshua David, God Danced the Day You Were Born." In smaller, black letters it read, "You are a gift to all mankind, His gift of love to them. You are His" (Richard Kramer, ND).

As I read the words aloud, my emotions surfaced, evidenced by my cracking voice and the tears cascading down my cheeks. My mother and I could not think of a more precious way to describe her first grandson's birth. God was bestowing a promise to Joshua that day, and these words have sustained us ever since.

Joshua ("Joshy") was a sweetheart of a baby. He was as pudgy as he was long. He ate ravenously and was quickly in the hundredth percentiles for height and weight. I couldn't resist squeezing and snuggling him every chance I had. His smile lit up the room and our hearts. All of his first year milestones were met with flying colors. Witnessing his first tooth, finding his thumb, sitting, and walking for the first time were all such a wonder to experience.

However, Joshy did not say his first word ("mama") until he was ten-months-old, which was a few months later compared to his sister. I ignored this minor blip on the developmental milestone chart because research showed that younger siblings tend to acquire human language slower, often because their older siblings communicate for them.

Alexa instantly fell in love with his chubby rolls and sweet laugh. I could often hear her whispering to him when he cried, "It's okay little buddy!" Alexa loved to feed him bottles and offer snuggles under their cozy blankies. She was becoming an excellent role model, big sister, and true friend to her little brother.

THE AIR I BREATHE

J oshua's health was precarious that first winter. He developed respiratory syncytial virus (RSV) which resulted in bronchiolitis and a three-day hospitalization. One afternoon as I changed his clothes on the diaper table, I watched his breathing become more labored. I was shocked to see blue lips, a concave chest, and a distended abdomen. I feared for his every breath.

Once I realized how dire the situation was, I called for Dave, and we jumped in the car, dismissing the safety and formality of the car seats. I clung to him against my chest with every ounce of love I could muster, and we raced to the Emergency Room. It was terrifying watching him listless in an isolation chamber, struggling for each breath. *Please Lord, let me breathe for him!* I thought. With proper medication, rest, and time, Joshy made a full recovery, but the disease left him susceptible to allergies and asthma.

The RSV scare catapulted us into a new territory filled with allergies, nebulizers, and eczema. For the next year, Joshy's cheeks were fiery red, scathed with an eczema rash. He wheezed with every cold and needed nebulizers filled with Pulmicort and Singulair. Six months into this regime, we took Joshy to a pediatric allergist. Sucking his thumb and holding blankie while nestled on my lap, he was pricked from head to toe for nearly an hour. He was also screaming his head off, confused as to why Mommy would let this nurse hurt him. My heavy heart wanted to take every twinge and prick on his behalf. The testing confirmed allergies to pollens, foods, dust, and molds. And this was only the tip of the iceberg.

FIRSTS

Joshy's first year of life was full of new beginnings. When he was nine-months-old, he was dedicated to the Lord. That day Dave and I promised to live under God's promises and instructions, and to dedicate our home and our son to the Lord. Dedication acknowledges what has already taken place in the heart. As parents, we committed to our God-given responsibility to maintain a Christian home, the center of which would be the Lord Jesus Christ, and to educate our children on Christian principals. That night I prayed over my sleeping angel, *"Lord, I am dedicating this precious baby to you. I pray you will bless his little life. Give our baby a heart to know you, a tender heart to love you always."*

During Joshy's first year of life, we decided this kid was going to see the world and go places! He spent countless hours enjoying the giraffe and swans at the Fort Wayne Children's Zoo. He went out on boat rides at the nearby lake, and took his first airplane trip to visit his grandparents in Connecticut. He also traveled to Cedar Point Amusement Park, in Sandusky Ohio, my favorite place to vacation when I was a child. Joshy was fascinated with the water park kiddie slides and sprinklers. He loved the sensation of sticking his head and arms into the cool streams of water. There was such contentment and joy during this trip; it seemed all was right with our world. It remains one of my fondest trips with the children.

With quality family time becoming a high priority, we started camping around Joshy's first birthday. Camping became such a wonderful way for us to enjoy nature and slow down the pace of our increasingly hectic lives. During Joshy's first camping trip at

Bear Creek Farms, he floated down his first lazy river, splashing gleefully at the water surrounding his floatie.

We also went to Chain O Lakes Campground where we strapped Joshy tightly in the hiking backpack atop his father's shoulders. He became an expert baby camper after completing this first hike. Joshy learned to walk in the great outdoors, pushing his walker through the dirt during the three days of torrential downpours at Jelly Stone Park. We found him face down in the mud a million times, but he always got back up and tried again. He was gaining his independence, and we could not have been more thrilled.

That stormy camping trip, the torrential downpours forced the frogs, worms, and insects inside our tent for refuge. I could hear Joshy's squeal of delight. "*Ogg, mama, ogg!*" Because of this up close and personal experience with wildlife, I vowed to never camp in a tent again. Wonderful as these initial camping experiences were, we left Jelly Stone Park, and I insisted Dave drive full speed ahead into an RV dealership to buy our first pop-up camper. Sleeping with frogs tested my limits. I was born and raised a city girl.

Another first for Joshy was an angelic intervention in his crib. One day after I put him down for a nap in his nursery, I ventured outside to get some yard work accomplished. Although Joshy usually slept for at least three hours, my intuition urged me to check on him after about one hour. When I approached the closed door to his bedroom, I quietly and carefully opened it. Surprised and alarmed, I rubbed my eyes to make sure I wasn't seeing things. There sat Joshua playing on the floor with a toy! *How could this be possible?*

My next glance was at the crib where I left him. It appeared my antique, Jenny Linn crib had seen its better days, as the hinges were broken off of the right corner. This made the bottom corner of the mattress pad and springs angle down lower than the rest of the frame. There was a slight possibility that Joshy's body could have wiggled through the small gap, but he wasn't walking yet. There was *no way* he could have gotten his head through the gap without getting choked. *How could he have climbed out and over the high crib walls?* Only an angel could have lifted up my baby and placed him unscathed onto the floor.

WORSHIP

Although life was getting busier with Alexa and Joshy, I still felt like I had my own identity. There was healthy balance between family, friends, motherhood, married life, and hobbies. I was able to work primarily from home by conducting personality assessments through a contract established with Goodwill Industries.

I also joined MOPS (Mothers of Preschoolers) at Blackhawk that fall. With a master's degree in counseling, stepping up into a leadership role for other young mothers was an opportunity for Christian community service. I organized activities, counseled young mothers, and provided encouragement and practical suggestions. I tried to become the poster child for parenting, and I pretended to have it all figured out on the outside. I loved these women but wondered if they could see my masquerade. *Can they see my true insecurities, Lord?*

I also ventured into the gift of music and song in 2001 by joining the Blackhawk Praise Team. While I spent my entire life having a love for song, I did not have much confidence in my abilities, nor had I sung publically to praise God. Yet here I found myself at twenty-seven years old, certain of three things.

1. I was blessed with the spiritual gift of harmony.
2. God was stretching my comfort zone.
3. It was time to openly express my devotion and love for the Lord.

I was moved by Scripture in Psalm 26:6-8 & 12 (NLT), which says,

I have come to your altar O Lord, singing a song of thanksgiving and telling of all your miracles. I love your sanctuary Lord, the place where your glory shines.....I have taken a stand, and I will publically praise the Lord!

I lived for the weekly practices and performances. Sometimes, however, Dave would get home late from work and have to meet me at church later than expected. On these nights, I had to haul the kids with me to church. As we warmed up before performances, Joshy would make such a racket that it embarrassed and distracted me. I was incredibly self conscious and so insecure.

Joshy had become inexplicably discontent, and I couldn't help but wonder if I was doing something wrong. I worried that others would judge my parenting skills. I wasn't ready to give up my masquerade of being a completely put-together, organized, deliriously happy mother of two little ones. I battled secret anxieties laced in self doubt. *Why do I care so much about what other people think about me, Lord? Why can't I focus only on pleasing you? Doesn't your Word encourage me to only to serve you?*

Despite Joshy's screaming and running around, the praise team was charmed with my exuberant son. Every so often, they allowed Joshy to come up on stage, grab a microphone, and sing his little heart out. His lips would press directly on the microphone, spreading graham cracker remnants and toddler drool. Initially Joshy could only create a muffled sound, but with persistence, loud, jubilant gibberish erupted. With either the hymnal or Holy Bible in hand, Joshy would lose himself while he sang. The melody was so pure and innocent being sung from the mouth of a babe! *So why is my joy tampered? Why am I always worried about his improper behavior rather than marveling at his angelic quality when he sings for the Lord?* I had much to learn in my walk with the Lord.

PRAISE YOU THROUGH THIS STORM

S tudying James 1:2-15 reminded me that God does not cause pain, but at times He allows me to be tested to increase my faithfulness. Verses 2-3 proclaim, "Consider it pure joy, my brothers and sisters, whenever you face trials of many kinds, because you know that the testing of your faith produces perseverance." I noticed that it did not say *if* I face trials. It says *when* I face trials. This was really good to know, because I had numerous trials hovering on the horizon.

After Joshy's birth, Dave accepted a new position at Depuy Orthopedics in Warsaw, Indiana. Although this was a forty minute commute, we opted to stay in Fort Wayne because we adored our local church community and friends. The job was a huge blessing for our family, but it required monthly travel as well as the daily commute. This left me home alone with the children more often, carrying my baggage of insecurities. A looming sense of inadequacy about my temperament as a mother was slowly creeping into the crevices of my self-esteem.

With Dave absent more often, I started feeling frustrated with Joshua's behavior as well as my reaction to his behavior. It seemed like nothing I tried worked. I was baffled. I counted to ten in a feeble attempt to be more patient. A simple cheek flick, hand swat, or time out did not faze him. The Christian parenting curriculum was *not* working. There was no educational method or disciplinary action that was impacting Joshy's behavior. *Why was it so simple with Alexa?*

An all-consuming, pervasive, melancholic affect swept over Joshy. He never seemed to grasp cause and effect and appeared confused by the consequences of his actions. Joshy ran around screaming and crying all day. I started to realize I had been given an adorable, curious, but extremely hyperactive little boy who was being driven by a motor from somewhere deep within. I realized that caring for him was turning into a triple-time job and that I had no time or energy left over for my work with Goodwill. Determined to focus all my energy on Joshy, I resigned from my position.

Luckily Dave and I agreed on naming our firstborn son Joshua, because we used every version of his name two thousand times daily. He simply did not respond or acknowledge his name. *Doesn't he understand his name? Is he ignoring us? Can he hear us?* I became so sick of repeating the very name we gave to our son whom we loved unconditionally. His name became heavy in my mouth, thickened with aggravation. The sounds would slough off my tongue as the six letters rolled out. "Joshua. Josh. Joshy! Joshuaaaaaaa!" People could see (and hear) my exasperation and fatigue because I was always calling his name and chasing him.

I spoke with Dave about my concerns with Joshy's intensity, constant crying, and high activity level. Unsure of how to proceed, we turned to the pediatrician. To our chagrin, she disregarded our concerns and surmised that the problem was our lack of experience at parenting, as "Joshy was just being a boy." How I hated that stereotype! Something in the depths of my heart told me otherwise. I felt so alone and misunderstood. *Why can't I make my son happy?*

In the spring of 2002, we finally decided to move to Warsaw so that Dave could have more family time and help with Joshua. The move offered us a period of hope and transition, a time for new beginnings, and the opportunity to find God's will for our lives. The positive mind shift and heart change I felt was a refreshing break from the despondency that had become my constant shadow in Fort Wayne.

THE GIFT OF FRIENDSHIP

I met her after living in Warsaw for one week. I had been praying for God to introduce me to a new friend, and there she waited at a McDonald's Play Land. Our daughters found each other in the jungle gym and then later introduced us. I eagerly chatted with this new woman holding her second-born, tiny baby girl in her arms. Her name was Christi, and she was meant to become my best friend overnight. I later learned that before she entered McDonald's that day, she fervently prayed that the Lord would place her on a path where she could make a difference and find significance in this world.

When we met inside the golden arches, we knew this was the beginning of a God-ordained friendship with Christ at the center. Uncanny coincidences bonded us that day:

1. We were born on the exact same day of the same year: September 26, 1972. (Who asks a stranger when her birthday is?)
2. We both had a deep love for Jesus. The Holy Spirit was covering us and encouraging us to expose some very personal details of ourselves.
3. We both had an intense passion for expressing our faith and emotions in creative ways. Both of us were ardent readers and writers. She was and continues to be a gifted artist and pianist, while I had a vehement affinity with music and song.

Initially, Christi was the only one who knew about my struggles with Joshua. She would wake early many mornings and be on her knees in prayer, humbly pleading with the Lord for my family to experience His mighty healing. She was living proof of the power of intercessory prayer; together we became a dynamic and effective spiritual duo.

Dave and I also met Chad and Mary the Stiver that year. I met Mary through the prayer group at church, and on a whim, I invited Mary and Chad to join us for a three day weekend getaway at French Lick Resort in southern Indiana. To my delight, they said yes! That memorable trip began the start of a wonderful friendship. Chad and Dave quickly became best friends, and Mary and I were thick as thieves.

There have been hearty laughs and amazing memories over the years, yet the most precious aspect of our friendship was our combined faith paired with the mutual struggles our sons endured. We found another family with which we could share our fears, discouragement, victories, and laughs. We were a safe haven for each other amidst the storms of life. Their friendship will always be invaluable to us.

EGG SHELLS

That fall we eagerly prepared for Alexa to attend Christian kindergarten at the Lutheran Church while Joshy would stay home with me. He occasionally attended the local preschool, but his behavior became increasingly difficult to manage. At home his tantrums were becoming longer, more volatile, and more self-injurious. The preschool also contacted me with similar concerns with his social skills, coping skills, and communication.

Joshy was like a light switch; one second he would be laughing, and the next, he would be incensed over something other children would find insignificant. He seemed rigid in his thinking, inflexible. There were no compromises. Naturally, I started walking on eggshells. Joshy's eggshells were unpredictable and very messy. I could never predict when an egg would break or the intense cleanup that it might require.

One time we were leaving home when somebody opened the door leading into the garage—no big deal. Yet to Joshy this was the end of the world as he knew it. Someone else's innocent action resulted in Joshy screaming bloody murder for twenty minutes. Joshy probably wanted to open the door himself, but he didn't have words to express that.

CAR RIDES

As a young mother, I had many errands to run, but the frequent car trips were like taking a ride down hell's highway. The screaming was relentless; Joshy hated being contained in his car seat. His long legs constantly kicked the back of my driver's seat, and he was always wailing. After enduring this for many months, I finally got creative and purchased industrial strength ear phones.

I knew it was not the safest driving option because I could not hear anything around me—not the traffic, the sirens, the radio, *or my children*. But that was the point, wasn't it? I convinced myself that it was safer to drive hearing impaired than with the continual distraction and chaos from my children. It was amazing how I could deceive myself when I was desperate. At the boyish age of two, Joshy always found a way to squirm out of his carseat. One cool, early spring morning I started the car to heat it up. I strapped Joshy into his seat, and quickly ran back inside to grab my purse. I couldn't have been gone for more than sixty seconds. In that time, my little Houdini had wiggled out from his five point harness system, climbed into the front seat and put the car in reverse. I walked out moments later to find my car slowly gliding down the driveway. I have never run so fast!

BEDROOM DRAMA

As Joshy's world became bigger, I tried to provide him with a peaceful bedroom for reading and sleeping. We must have had five hundred books to peruse. Every night, when I tucked him safely into his covers, the books were nestled into their special shelves and drawers. But my little guy was such an opportunist! He simply could not resist playing with them in the wee hours of the morning before the rest of us awoke. Joshy was developing an affinity for books—but not for reading. Instead, he was obsessed with ripping the pages and throwing each and every one onto the floor. My hard work was his delight because his fun resulted in special time with mommy singing Barney's "Clean Up Song"!

I also created a mural on Joshy's blue bedroom walls, hoping I could create a sense of safety and relaxation. Inspired by Christi's artwork, I painted a scene with trains coming through mountains while nebulous, puffy, white clouds wafted by. Unfortunately, this gentle, quiet ambience did nothing to derail Joshy's nighttime fears. He clung to me for dear life at bedtime; many nights he woke up screaming from graphic nightmares that his limited language could hardly describe.

To empower him through those nights, I manufactured my very own "angel spray" to soothe him. These were merely aerosol cans of room deodorizer decorated with love by mom. Every evening I would spread my arms wide, turn a slow circle, and spray throughout the room while citing this simple prayer I learned as a child, "Angel of God my guardian dear, to whom God's love entrusts me here, forever this day be at my side, to lead and guard, to light and guide" (Richert, 2011).

Sometimes I sent Joshy his room to calm down, though it was never effective. He would hide behind the glider rocker, crying endlessly. He had not developed any strategies for calming himself other than sucking his thumb. I have one of these incidents on videotape. Part of my rationale for videotaping was that most of his misbehavior was reserved for me alone. This was my proof to show others that I was not losing my mind. Although I shared the video with Dave, neither of us has ever wanted to watch it again because it exposed our fractured family. The house was trashed, Joshy was crazed, and I was desperate to console my son.

STARTING TO MAKE SENSE

When Joshy turned two, I remember praying to God that this very day was going to be the start of a better year. I discovered a nonprofit program, The Cardinal Center, which offered assistance for young children with behavior and developmental delays. (Later I recognized this program as an early intervention service for children with special needs.) We were so excited the morning of the home assessment. *Can they possibly help my son?* I thought. When a kind, female evaluator greeted us at the door, Joshy immediately warmed up to her. He was on cloud nine because he had her immediate, individual attention.

Joshy was very compliant that day, which concerned me because I feared his "true colors" wouldn't show. It's not that I wanted my son to have something wrong, but I yearned to find a problem they could fix. The evaluator conducted multiple assessments to evaluate his communication, behavior, fine motor, visual perceptual, and sensory processing skills. To my dismay, my primary areas of concern—communication and behavior—only indicated minor delays, which did not qualify him for services.

However, the occupational therapy assessment was interesting if not alarming. At one point during the evaluation Joshy had the luxury of playing with shaving cream on foil. This activity provided instant pleasure; the evaluator said she had never seen such an extreme reaction to the "messy art." Not only did Joshy rub his hands throughout the shaving cream, but he smothered it all over his face, body, and clothes.

It appeared like Joshy wanted more of the good feeling the shaving cream yielded. He searched desperately for more of that smooth, cool, calming sensation. He couldn't get enough! He looked like a snowman when the bottle went dry. This light-hearted assessment revealed that Joshy had atypical auditory processing, visual processing, vestibular processing, and oral sensory processing. It was official; she labeled Joshy as having a sensory processing disorder. This meant it was difficult for Joshy to regulate his body and emotions in response to the input he received from his environment.

Ultimately the Cardinal Center refused to qualify him for services based on a sensory processing disorder because he did not have another "significant delay" according to their standards. As a consolation prize, the evaluator recommended I purchase the book *The Out-of-Sync Child* (Kranowitz, 1998) which described sensory processing disorders. I was encouraged to focus on portions dedicated to having a "sensory seeking child."

I bought that darned book. Despite my initial reluctance, it quickly became a valid resource that helped me understand how my son's brain worked. I learned that as a "sensory seeker," Joshy's body was under-responsive to many senses. Joshy could not register tactile senses (touch) accurately, so he did not feel pain as acutely as others. He also required deep pressure to calm down. Joshy did not feel food on his face, filthy hands, or bruised knees. Joshy also craved physical activity—the more bouncing and running, the better! Furthermore, he was unaware of his body in space (proprioception), which impacted his balance. He was constantly falling down, bumping into things, and bruised from head to toe.

However, in other ways, Joshy was a "sensory avoider," meaning he was overstimulated by other sensory input at different times. For example, he despised being cold and hated the snow. The cold air felt like a billion stinging needles pricking his delicate skin. I tried to force him to enjoy the outdoors with his sister as I dressed him in thick snow gear. The poor kid was immobilized in his snowsuit like the little boy from *A Christmas Story* (Clark, 1983).

Forcing him to play outside bundled in a snowsuit is a great example of how difficult it was for me to see the world from his viewpoint. I embraced new experiences with eagerness and excitement. Exploring new situations and my environment has always been a rewarding and positive experience. However, Joshy had no desire to try anything new that involved changes in activity, temperature, sound, or sensation. The discomfort and fear he experienced was simply too much to bear. The everyday experiences I took for granted became terrifying and dreadful prospects for Joshy.

My frame of reference for what I considered to be pleasant activities extended from my personality and life experiences. It was challenging to not get discouraged with worry that life was passing him by because he didn't want to do anything I considered fun. *Lord, please help me achieve a balance between accepting Joshy's sensory problems and nudging him gently beyond his comfort zone*, I prayed.

Crowds and constant loud noises were also overstimulating, resulting in meltdowns. Joshy wanted to crawl under a table and hide from these activities. He was inconsolable during parades; nothing soothed him. Hands covering his ears and screaming, Joshy must have heard the sirens at the decibel a dog can hear. Changes in routine, environment, and transitions were also overwhelming for his system. He didn't seem to have the ability to make sense of the changes in the world around him, and his body could not adapt or assimilate accordingly.

Armed with new insight on what made Joshy tick, I went on a shopping spree to purchase therapeutic toys. There is a world of amazing therapeutic toys for children out there! Occupational therapy (OT) gifts were a staple that year for his birthday and Christmas. Joshy received an electric toothbrush to increase oral stimulation, chew toys, and a bouncy ball for proprioceptive regulation. OT toys were the hit of every celebration!

ALPHABET SOUP

S ince the intensity and duration of Joshy's tantrums were getting worse, Dave and I decided it was time to take him to a therapist. We still did not know what to attribute his mood swings and hyperactivity to, and frankly, we needed help. After one session with Joshy, the therapist looked us in the eye and in his monotone voice he stated, "Joshy either has attention deficit hyperactivity disorder (ADHD), early onset bipolar disorder, or both." We were stunned. The hairs bristled on my arms, and my mother bear claws came out in effort to protect Joshy from the bad names the therapist called him. I could understand an ADHD diagnosis, but bipolar disorder? *Really? Joshy is so very young, Lord!* I thought.

I boasted of my own credentials in the mental health field. I refused to acknowledge the possibility of a mood imbalance. It's ironic how all of my credentials and professional experience could not prepare me for a professional's opinion on why my son was struggling. While I knew there was something abnormal (I use that term loosely), the affirmation from the clinician ripped another tiny piece of my heart away. It made it real. Legitimate. He had officially been diagnosed with ADHD and Sensory Processing Disorder.

I went home and pulled out my dusty second bible from graduate school, *The Diagnostic and Statistical Manual of Mental Disorders* (DSM-IV) (American Psychiatric Association, 2000). The DSM-IV affirms that either category number one or category number two must be present to meet criteria for ADHD.

I. Six or more of the following symptoms of inattention have been present for at least six months to a point that is disruptive and inappropriate for developmental level:

1. (one) Inattention:

    (a) Often does not give close attention to details or makes careless mistakes in schoolwork, work, or other activities. (check)
    (b) Often has trouble keeping attention on tasks or play activities. (check)
    (c) Often does not seem to listen when spoken to directly. (check)
    (d) Often does not follow instructions and fails to finish schoolwork, chores, or duties in the workplace (not due to oppositional behavior or failure to understand instructions). (check)
    (e) Often has trouble organizing activities. (check)
    (f) Often avoids, dislikes, or doesn't want to do things that take a lot of mental effort for a long period of time (such as schoolwork or homework). (check)
    (g) Often loses things needed for tasks and activities (e.g. toys, school assignments, pencils, books, or tools). (check)
    (h) Is often easily distracted. (check)
    (i) Is often forgetful in daily activities. (check)

II. Six or more of the following symptoms of hyperactivity-impulsivity have been present for at least six months to an extent that is disruptive and inappropriate for developmental level:

1. (one) Hyperactivity:

(a) Often fidgets with hands or feet or squirms in seat. (check)

(b) Often gets up from seat when remaining in seat is expected. (check)

(c) Often runs about or climbs when and where it is not appropriate (adolescents or adults may feel very restless). (check)

(d) Often has trouble playing or enjoying leisure activities quietly. (check)

(e) Is often "on the go" or often acts as if "driven by a motor." (check)

(f) Often talks excessively. (check)

2. (two) Impulsivity:

(a) Often blurts out answers before questions have been finished. (check)

(b) Often has trouble waiting one's turn. (check)

(c) Often interrupts or intrudes on others (e.g., butts into conversations or games). (check)

Furthermore, some symptoms must be before age seven years and manifest in two or more settings (e.g. at school/work and at home). There must also be clear evidence of significant impairment in social, school, or work functioning. Finally, the symptoms do not happen only during the course of a pervasive developmental disorder, schizophrenia, or other psychotic disorder, and they are not better accounted for by another mental disorder (e.g. mood disorder, anxiety disorder, dissociative disorder, or a personality disorder).

Okay, fine….fair enough. The evidence was staring at me in the face. Joshy most certainly met criteria for ADHD.

SHRINKING

The family therapist referred Joshy to his first psychiatrist—actually, it was the only psychiatrist in our small town. Dr. Romboldi was willing to treat Joshy's hyperactivity with a small dose of the stimulant Ritalin. Never in my wildest imagination did I think I would be electively medicating my two-year-old; the guilt was unbearable. *If I was a better mother...If I had more patience...If I wouldn't have let the doctor induce his labor two years ago...If I...* Although I temporarily stifled my guilt when I saw the benefit Ritalin had on reducing Joshy's hyperactivity and impulsivity, my own relief never lasted long. I was always waiting for the other shoe to drop, expecting something bad to happen. And when it did, the guilt returned with a vengeance.

After two weeks on Ritalin, I started to notice the first of many side effects he was to endure. Although Ritalin quieted down Joshy's internal motor, he started to have mind-boggling mood swings lasting all day and evening. His only relief was sleep. There was this intensity—a persistent ferocity—an irritability in navigating relationships and understanding limitations. After enduring a few months of these pervasive, extreme mood swings, I started to worry. *Perhaps the family therapist was correct...does he have an underlying mood disorder?* The stimulants were making him better in one way, yet hurting him in other ways.

Although I've blocked out most of these painful memories, family videos remind me how drastically my house was falling apart. My house was filthy with clothing scattered in every room; dishes were strewn across all countertops. I didn't have time or energy to bother, and my emotions were worn thin. I lost all self-esteem as a mother.

For someone who loved being in control, there was nothing about this situation that resembled a peaceful, controlled, harmonious existence. At follow up appointments with the psychiatrist, I found myself swinging to the other side of the pendulum, begging for help for with Joshy's mood. But Dr. Romboldi refused to address my concerns regarding Joshy's mood instability. Instead, we were the "lucky" recipients of her sympathy prescription Clonidine (typically used for blood pressure regulation), which did nothing more than sedate him and give him diarrhea. Joshy slept constantly. *What kind of life is this for a little boy? I'm drugging my boy. God help me,* I thought.

Despite the chaos and trepidation I felt for my son's future, God lifted me up during these days. I had nearly every verse in Philippians 4 highlighted in yellow. Closest to my heart were verses 6-7; they carried me through the worst hours:

> Do not be anxious in anything, but in everything, by prayer and petition, present your requests to God. And the peace that transcends all understanding will guard your hearts and your minds in Christ Jesus.

Amen. *That's what I'm counting on Lord.*

MEDICAL MYSTERY NUMBER ONE

Joshy was a few months shy of his second birthday when one unsuspecting morning he developed a severe case of hives. I was concerned because he was crying, itching, and feverish as well. I took him to the Kosciusko Community Hospital's Emergency Room, fearing he was having some sort of allergic reaction. But the doctors could not find a cause, so they sent him home on the steroid Prelone and antihistamines to reduce inflammation. If only it would have been that simple.

The hives disappeared the next day, but the day after, they reappeared with a vengeance. Our second trip to the emergency room resulted in the same treatment plan: "Go home, rest, take steroids and antihistamines. Good luck." I became skeptical of the doctor's impressions, believing they truly didn't care; I knew they would forget us the second we left. But Joshy wasn't getting any better.

The sun set then rose one more time when I awoke to piercing screams echoing down the hallway. It was a scream of agony. I rushed into Joshy's bedroom to find him shaking under the covers, his face scrunched in pain. Frantic, he cried out that he was unable to move his legs. I tried to help him stand, but his little legs crumbled in weakness and pain. There was a lacey rash covering his body, hives, and his temperature was 102 degrees. These symptoms were not characteristic of a typical childhood illness such as chicken pox or fifth's disease. I could not fathom what was wreaking havoc inside his sensitive little body.

One million worst case scenarios flooded my apprehensive mind.

I responded on auto pilot. First I called my mother in Ohio and asked her to rush over to Indiana to get Alexa before she was released from school that afternoon. In the meantime, I headed to the pediatrician, *not* the emergency room. This time the pediatrician took one look at my little lamb and agreed that enough was enough. She ordered him to be admitted to Lutheran Hospital in Fort Wayne. Joshua stayed in the hospital for two and a half days with inexplicable joint pain, fever, and rash. His blood work revealed a high white blood cell count of seventeen thousand. His little body was definitely fighting an ominous something.

Joshy's symptoms were a medical mystery. The nurses encouraged him to attempt standing on his legs, but medical records indicated his reluctance Saying, "Joshua was screaming when we tried to make him stand up." Even the doctors saw the agony in his eyes. They documented, "He cries when he looks at me...but he can be comforted by his parents, which is good."

After another day of observation, the team administered another oral dose Prelone when finally his fever broke. Slowly the rash and hives disappeared and his mobility returned. Joshy was released with prescriptions for the antibiotic Zithromax and allergy medications including Zyrtec and Singulair. The medicine was the equivalent of placing a thin band aid over a gushing wound. It served only as a small patch meant to repair the problem for a minute, without ever discovering the root cause.

The doctor's best guess was that Joshy either had an allergic reaction, a virus, or something vague called "serum sickness." Serum sickness is a hypersensitive reaction that occurs in response to certain antiserums. The body's immune system mistakes a protein in the antiserum as an antigen, and white blood cells attack it. The body then develops an immune response against the antiserum (Serum Sickness, 2011). Ten thousand dollars later, this vague, disappointing explanation did not make sense to me. That's the medical system working for you.

MY BUTTERFLY

There were endless days and nights where all my focus and attention went into parenting Joshy. Medication distributions, behavior management, and chasing him constantly for ten hours each day exhausted me. Mercifully, sweet slumber captured Joshy's body and mind around seven each night.

The evenings became what I dubbed "special time" for Alexa. At four-years-old, she was growing up before my eyes and before her time. I felt her childhood slipping away as she took on more independence and responsibilities than her age required. With the bittersweet realization that my butterfly would one day fly far, far away, I resolved to make our evenings full of fun and laughter.

Alexa and I really cherished our special time together. We laid in bed together reading *I Spy* books and traced letters on each other's backs. We shared stories, laughter, and love, just the two of us. During those evenings when Alexa felt most safe, she started asking questions about her brother. Why did the Lord let him cry all the time? Why was he always in trouble? My heart crumbled at her questions. We prayed together that someday Joshy would be healed. I prayed that this situation would not turn Alexa away from God, but instead that He would use her experience to bring glory to His name.

SUGAR AND BLANKIES

J oshy's second birthday quickly approached. The day he blew out the candles on his Thomas the Train birthday cake I fervently prayed, *"Lord, please let this be the first day of a better year for Joshy and our family. Please!"*

It took me those first two years to learn that I had to meet Joshy where he was at, not where I wanted him to be. For example, I wanted to document Joshy's momentous second birthday with none other than a Walmart photograph. I knew he would never sit still for the picture, so my sneaky little mind concocted a plan. I knew I had to plan, coordinate, and downright manipulate the situation in order to make this mission successful.

We went to Walmart with my secret arsenal in tow. Imagine Joshy's delight when he arrived and found his favorite blue, tug boat toy, blankie, and best of all—*candy*! I placed Joshy inside the tugboat, wrapped his blankie around him, and bribed him with red jelly beans. The first picture captured his glee perfectly. Mission accomplished.

The jelly beans worked their magic because back at home, Joshy started to have intense sugar cravings. The intensity of the cravings was worse than any child's occasional desire for a Popsicle. It always escalated into relentless begging, crying, and yanking on my legs in desperation nearly every fifteen minutes. Treats preoccupied his mind; he often thought of nothing else except when he could get his next sugar fix.

Joshy also became quite attached to his blankie as many toddlers do. Unfortunately, we had to replace his precious blankie due to safety hazards. How many other children's lives were in peril due to an innocent blankie? The evidence spoke for itself. We found white lint balls following his path wherever he went. Joshy developed a fascination with picking fuzzies off the blanket material. He would obsessively shove them up his nose as a way to self comfort. Creative coping mechanism, yes. Safe behavior, no!

Despite my best efforts at managing my family, everything seemed so out of my control. I knew it was not my responsibility to control everyone and everything, so I prayed for God's help daily. Yet I still struggled to resist the temptation to jump in and take charge of all things external. I found myself challenging God. *I know what's best for my son. That's why you gave him to me, right Lord?* I became a gatekeeper, judiciously either permitting or denying certain influences in my son's life. I was cautious with the medical community, television shows, music, fellow brothers and sisters in Christ, and even my family. I felt like although they all wanted to help and support me, they could not truly understand the life we were living.

I believed nobody could understand how lonely and scared I felt; it was a sinking, desperate feeling. I understood that the Lord placed certain supports in my life for a reason, yet the more out of control life spun, the stronger I resisted the help. I felt like if I accepted other's mercy and grace, that it was my resignation to weakness. I obviously had a difficult time surrendering control to God, which in hindsight is ironic because shepherding this family was never mine to control anyway.

My need to relinquish control and give it all up the Lord is a recurrent theme I have wrestled with my entire life. But He won't give up on me. I'll get there someday.

PUPPY LOVE

For a mother with control issues, it was completely illogical to add another wildcard to the mix, but I did it anyway. I am a huge sucker for animals—especially cats and dogs. One day I found (okay, I searched for) a soft, fuzzy puppy who won over my heart. We named her Sadie. She was a beautiful, gentle Sheltie puppy—a miniature Lassie hero with whom Joshy formed a special connection. Their affinity toward one another was beautiful. Joshy's relationship with Sadie became the first of many special animals in his life.

Through Sadie, we had discovered another unique and lovely gift that God granted my son—a special kinship with animals. Sadie and Joshy comforted each other without words; they communicated effortlessly with simple gestures. Sadie's presence calmed Joshy. When he was unable to find coping mechanisms within him, Sadie was an excellent substitution. Through their friendship, Joshy's kindness and gentleness became more transparent to everyone.

ALL ABOARD

After the excitement over Sadie's adoption dissipated and the holidays had passed, the winter doldrums set in. Thankfully Dave has recognized over the years that if his wife is happy, then the family is happy. He generously agreed to boost my spirits with a little Caribbean sunshine, and my spirit delighted in the idea of a family vacation.

We decided to take a last minute cruise with the two children to the Virgin Islands. It was spontaneous and relatively inexpensive, and my mind began to weave together huge expectations of the perfect family experience. *Life is so difficult at home, this vacation must be exactly what you want us to do Lord!* Or not. There were only two things about that vacation that Joshy liked:

1. (one) The towel animals placed on his bed every night.
2. (two) The food.

Otherwise, you could find him miserable, inconsolable, and crying.

Although the cruise ship's Kids Corner program enabled parents to have some much needed quality time alone, they wouldn't allow Joshy to stay because he was still in diapers. The only exception to him staying, they explained, would be for his sister to change him. So at the tender age of five, Alexa was introduced to her first babysitting lesson: poopy diapers 101. Bless her heart; she was so excited to take care of her little brother—ready, willing, and able. Dave and I prayed whenever the kids went to the daycare. *Lord, please, please, please don't let Joshy poop while he's at Kids Corner! Can you just stop this one biological function for a few hours each day?* Luckily God heard our pleas because Alexa's duties were never needed.

Dinners were horrific. The couple that shared our dinner table every night had to endure the exhaustion and tears right along with us. We felt so terrible for this other family trying to have a relaxing meal. Joshy fell asleep every night with his head on the tray by seven. Toward the end of the cruise, I sat back and asked the heavy weighted question looming over my head and piercing my heart. *Lord, what exactly is wrong with my son?* He couldn't handle being in a new environment. Everything seemed to scare him and make him cry. There was no sparkle or joy behind his eyes. When somebody you love is that miserable, it is difficult to relax and have your own good time. My perfect vacation was devastated. Shattered.

We returned from our voyage exhausted, but with more determination than ever before to find out if Joshy really did have bipolar disorder.

THE LAST FRENCH FRY

The more I learned about bipolar disorder, I emphatically believed Joshy met the criteria. Although diagnosing a child with bipolar was controversial, Joshy's symptoms were blatant.

He nearly possessed all the characteristics described for other children with bipolar disorder. He struggled with separation anxiety, night terrors, oppositional behavior, difficulty with sensory processing, raging, rapid cycling, difficulty with peer relationships, bedwetting, cravings for carbohydrates and sweets, and overreactions to hot and cold. Joshy also lived in mixed emotional states. This is an emotional episode that simultaneously presents symptoms of both depression and mania (Dimitri Papolos M.D. & Janice Papolos, 1999/2006).

Joshy endured marked agitation, constant restlessness, high energy, self-destructiveness, and sadness *every day of his life*. I could see the misery behind his eyes and how scared he was of his own rage. After 95 percent of Joshy's rages, when the light switch suddenly turned off, he would burst into tears, hugging me, pleading with me to forgive him. He literally could not squelch the rage.

Joshy was always extremely remorseful, because his heart really only wanted to please his mommy and daddy. Often Joshy would ask me, "Why am I a bad boy, Mommy?" and together we would melt into tears as I reassured him, "Joshy, you are a *good* boy. A sweet, loving, good boy." Throughout the years this cycle has continued. If he lost control over his behavior and emotions, the self-hate, guilt, and shame permeated over his heart. He was always heartbroken by his outbursts.

One day I took Joshy with me to meet my girlfriend Mary at the McDonald's Play Land. It was time to leave, and Joshy was already irritable because he received his five minute warning before it was time to leave. After all, he did *not* want to leave such an exciting place! To ease the transition (otherwise known as bribery) I bought him a small French fry. He was happy as a clam while I carried him outside toward the car. But as we crossed the pavement, the unthinkable happened… a few of his french fries fell onto the black parking lot. This was a colossal catastrophe for Joshy who quickly became inconsolable.

When he could not stop the kicking and screaming after ten minutes, something inside me snapped. I emphatically told Mary, "I will find that psychiatrist today while Joshy is in this state of mind. Nothing will stop me!" I called Dr. Romboldi's office but the receptionist stated she was working in another town over an hour away. I begged for that facility's number. I finally convinced them to share her contact information, and I called the facility to plead with them to see Joshy immediately because this was an emergency.

The secretary could not promise an appointment but allowed me to start driving there. In the meantime, my heart was racing; I was overflowing with anxiety and anticipation. Two hands gripped the steering wheel as I pierced the speed limit on back country roads. Joshy continued to screech in the back seat, and for once in my life I actually prayed for him to *continue* the behavior.

Of course he quieted down five minutes prior to our arrival. *Dang! Come on, act up kid!* I dragged him into the office and with tears in my eyes, begged them to let me in. They must have felt either compassion or pity for me because they quickly led us to a room. Initially Joshy appeared content with Dr. Romboldi. I, however, was freaking out inside, dying for Joshy to validate my description of his mood instability.

And then it happened. A simple no did the trick. Joshy was being destructive, ripping up magazines when he heard that nasty, forbidden word—no. He flipped out. He screamed, wailed, kicked, threw magazines, tossed chairs, and hid under the furniture. After this fifteen minute tirade (she was lucky it was so short!), she took one hard look at me and said, "Your son has bipolar disorder."

I didn't care about the diagnosis at that time as much as I cared about the treatment. I wanted him to have peace in his world. We both craved relief from this madness. Dr. Romboldi sent us on our way with a prescription of Risperdal, an atypical anti-psychotic which aides in mood stabilization. The description of this pill terrified me. *Anti-psychotic. Does that mean he's crazy?* I received samples in the office, and before my car left the parking lot, Joshy had his first dose.

Within ten minutes I felt the world's axis settle gently into place as a peace permeated the car—Joshy fell asleep. Sweet relief. By the time we returned home, this child of mine was downright pleasant for the next five hours. I slept fitfully that night, believing that our day not only held answers with a new diagnosis, but also for a treatment plan to thwart those ugly mood swings.

CHILDHOOD DAZE

There still were joyous moments entrenched between the tough times. Joshy loved visiting Cedar Point's water park, Soak City. We also made cross country trips with our camper to Hershey Park, and we traveled to Connecticut to see Dave's parents. Toys became quite impressionable at this age. Joshy's interests were with John Deere tractors, Buzz Light Year, matchbox cars, Tickle Me Elmo's, Thomas the Train, rider toys, noisy toys. He also spent endless afternoons allowing Alexa to torture him by dressing him up as a girl and playing kitchen.

As I watched Joshy play, I started to realize that he could not sustain his attention to a preferred activity for more than two minutes. I also noticed that his sleep patterns were sporadic and often interrupted by snoring. I started to wonder if his inattention and volatile moods were related to sleep deprivation. A trip to the local ENT doctor confirmed a diagnosis of enlarged tonsils and adenoids which could only to be corrected with surgery. Joshy's recovery from the procedure was excruciating, but it was a perfect opportunity to lavish some extra TLC his way. After two weeks of healing, the snoring was officially gone, but Joshy continued to wake up frequently during the night.

Caring for a toddler with special medical and behavioral needs left me exhausted and irritable. Frequently I sought counsel from my mother over the telephone; she provided me with encouragement and strength to move forward each day. However, one particular occasion I shared my frustrations with my father instead. At first I was reticent to share my struggles with him because he had his own sickness and anxieties. But ultimately, I knew he loved me dearly and felt great compassion for Joshy.

After I confided to my father about what a difficult time I was having, he generously offered to send Joshy to a private day care a few days each week. The goal was to provide me with some relief from his constant demands, as well as encourage his socialization skills. Although Joshy loved going to the daycare, he had difficulty interacting with other children. He was extremely emotional, prone to temper tantrums, and had limited communication skills. *Why does he have to struggle, Lord? Please bless him with friendships and peace.*

Although I had already been struggling with Joshy's behaviors for nearly two years, Dave was often working so he was not privy to Joshy's intensity. But on Easter 2003, reality sunk in for Dave. That morning Dave attempted to dress Joshy and fix the belt on the adorable Easter outfit he chose for this special occasion. Across the house Alexa and I rummaged through her Easter basket overflowing with candy while we listened to Joshy's familiar screaming back in the bedroom. *Hmm...they've been back there for over twenty minutes.* I started wondering if everything was alright.

Finally, when Dave came out frustrated beyond belief, I saw the foreboding fear in his eyes for the first time. The dreaded question transmitted wordlessly between us. "Why does everything have to be so difficult with this child?"

THE ITCH

The itch was setting in again. Joshy was enjoying some relief from the mood swings, and I was getting a break while he went to daycare for a few hours each week. Thoughts and visions swirled through my head day and night. *Is this for real? Do I actually have that burning desire once again to bring another life into this world? How can I possibly want another child? As if my hands aren't full enough, Lord!*

I tried to ignore the urge, but it wouldn't go away. I prayed for months before I approached Dave that winter. The prompting I felt to have a third child was so insane—completely illogical! Since there was nothing practical or convenient about expanding our family, I believed it was the Lord's will, and we were to trust in Him.

Dave and I served as worship leaders at a marriage retreat that February when we conceived our third child. I was over the moon! I fervently prayed this final addition to our clan would be another girl. Patience was never my virtue, so in true fashion, I inquired about the gender during an ultrasound. I claimed I wanted to know the gender because it was practical, and so I could be prepared. But secretly, I really just wanted to brace myself for the terrifying reality that this could be a boy.

I've tried to understand why I was so desperate to have another girl. It was complicated. I grew up with one sister and only played with my female cousins. I held onto visions that I would have two daughters with a close relationship like Jessica and me. I was naïve and ignorant; I didn't think it was possible for brothers to achieve that same special bond. I didn't understand boys, and if Joshua's trials were a template for raising these little chaps, then

I was signing on the dotted line for another girl. That summer I was especially vulnerable to Satan. He planted bad seeds in my heart and negative thoughts in my mind. He did not want me to experience the absolute joy of raising another little boy.

My high hopes were squashed when I realized I was indeed having another boy as the words, "See the turtle?" sunk in. I was devastated. Quickly, the devastation was replaced with self-loathing. I wondered how I could be such a despicable person to feel this way. *Lord, how could you do this to me? How can I handle two little Joshua's?*

Joshua was beautiful inside and out; he was a child of God. But he took all my energy, and I was overwhelmed. I am ashamed to admit this, but I cried for three days. I was terrified of the genetic lottery, the unknown, the "what ifs." If only my faith was as big as the mustard seed Jesus refers to in His Word:

> Jesus replied "I tell you the truth, if you have faith as small as a mustard seed, you can say to this mountain, 'Move from here to there' and it will move. Nothing will be impossible for you.
>
> —Matthew 17:20

The next day I marched down the road to Pastor Berry's house. He and his wife answered the door and found me standing there with tears in my eyes. I challenged biblical wisdom as I spewed forth Psalm 37: 3-4 (ESV). "Pastor Berry, the Bible says, 'Trust in the Lord, and do good; dwell in the land and befriend faithfulness. Delight yourself in the Lord, and he will give you the desires of your heart.' I know God wants to grant us the deepest desires of our hearts. So you tell me *why am I having another son?*"

Pastor Berry helped me realize I was interpreting the scripture only in a way that suited my emotions in the moment and that I had failed to acknowledge the other directives in those passages. My fear of the future far outweighed my trust in the Lord. And I certainly was not dwelling in the land of faithfulness and delight! I wanted the blessing described at the end of the passage without following the Lord's instructions. Pastor Berry offered encouragement by sharing Romans 8:28 (NASB), "And we know that God causes all things to work together for good to those who love God, to those who are called according to His purpose." I clung to this promise for dear life.

THIRD BIRTHDAY LETTER

My precious little boy, what a year you have had! One of such struggles and blessings, one of such growth. Although you have had some difficult times this past year with your behavior and health, those times have made me love you even more. You are so special. God gave you as a gift to us for a reason. Not so that we can "help" you, but so that you can teach us about life and how Jesus wants us to raise you and encourage us to be good examples to you. You have taught me so much this year. Patience (never enough!), unconditional love, the resilience and innocence of children, and that God answers prayers. There are many sweet things I think of when I remember you being two…

I see a little boy who is the tallest on the block! As your birthday has loomed closer I have loved seeing the curls starting to sprout all over your beautiful head. It's just like Mommy's hair grew when she was your age. I see the most exuberant boy in the morning, just ready to embrace the day. Some of your favorite things have been Jay Jay the Jet Plane and Thomas the Train. Your favorite song has been "I've Been Working on the Railroad," which you insisted I sing every night at bedtime. And now you love to sing—it is so precious! Your favorite book (which you ripped but are getting a new one for your birthday) is "Everyone Poops." You are so funny. Daddy just started working on your baseball swing and you just may have the knack! Now golf is a different story. You kind of look like a hockey player when you try to swing—it's so cute.

You are so excited to start preschool this fall, and you copy everything Alexa does. Did you know you already have five cavities due to your obsession with candy? We need to brush better this year! Nobody can ever replace you, Joshy. You pray with the sweetest spirit—eyes closed and focusing on that prayer. Your enthusiasm is contagious. Your cheesy smile is adorable. You are the love of our lives and will be the best big brother to baby Caleb in November. Joshy, you are beautifully and wonderfully made. Never forget that God danced the day you were born!

Love always,
Mommy

FIRE STARTER

As my pregnancy progressed, many anticipated expenses loomed upon the horizon. *The diapers! The clothing! The college education!* I wanted to contribute financially to the family, but by the same token, I didn't want to give up being at home with the kids. With money on my mind, I began to train for a career in home based medical transcription. I was so excited to be able to have an income while staying at home and taking care of my babies. I started the work with enthusiasm, but I was quickly reminded that I could never take a break from one true calling—Joshy. My eyes needed to stay on him at *all* times!

Whenever I started typing, the focus was taken off Joshy and the house became disturbingly quiet. The Tickle Me Elmo DVD's could only pacify him for so long. The unnatural quiet alerted my senses that trouble was brewing. One afternoon I was typing and enjoying the sweet smell of my "Home Sweet Home" Yankee Candle. As I enjoyed the calming scent lingering throughout the house, quietness suddenly saturated the air. *Bad sign.* I rushed to the kitchen and to my dismay, there sat Joshy sitting on top of the table, wafting napkins into the candle's open flame. I quit transcription the following week. It was either that or throw out the candles.

Joshy's activity level and curiosity persisted, resulting in another fire setting incident. One time he and his sister were playing in the basement with a toy broom when he stuck it into the fireplace where it inadvertently caught on fire. When Alexa started screaming Joshy became terrified. He waved the flaming broomstick wildly through the air, and then slammed it to the ground, creating patches of fire on the carpet. Quickly we extinguished the fire; praise God nobody was injured and our home was left standing! While Joshy didn't do these things intentionally, it seemed his impulsivity and complete disregard for safety made him a danger to himself and others.

CALEB "BOO" THOMAS

Caleb was born on October 31, 2003, two weeks before my due date. At dinnertime Dave and I left a confused, chubby cheeked, big, blue M&M and a beautiful, forlorn bumblebee on my front porch steps with empty pumpkins. Although I was heading to the hospital to give birth on Halloween, my young ones were understandably upset as they peered down into their empty baskets. Their mission for chocolates and candies was thwarted by Caleb's entrance into this world. That night the Lord blessed me Caleb Thomas Bierut. I immediately nicknamed my Halloween baby "Boo." I finally felt like my family was complete, and I truly loved all three of my darlings equally. Joshy was exceptionally tender with his baby brother. Caleb brought renewed hope for the future for all of us.

After Caleb's birth clarity washed over me. I finally understood that the Lord brought me Caleb because He needed to teach me He was the only one in the driver's seat. The Lord knew what was best for me. He brought me another son who has showed me just how much love and joy little boys can truly bring their mothers.

GROCERY MAYHEM

Caring for three children ages five and under was rewarding but challenging. Especially difficult were the times that required me to take all three of them out to run errands. I dreaded my weekly trip to the supermarket because there was nothing peaceful about the experience. One time I had all three children with me as I attempted to hunt and gather for my brood. Caleb's car seat took up half the cart, but we forged onward with Joshy crouched in the back between the diapers, fruits snacks, and cereals. Shopping for food was always precarious because the two oldest children constantly begged for sweets and snacks.

This particular day, everything climaxed at the checkout aisle when Joshy made his umpteenth request for a sucker. But when he heard no for the millionth time, it catapulted him into a screaming tailspin. He writhed on the dirty cement floor, kicking and flailing his little body. Everybody gawked at my very own Tasmanian devil twirling on the ground. I wanted to pick all of their jaws off the floor and throw them in a dumpster. I was mortified.

I never purchased the food that day, as the need to remove Joshy from the store proved most imminent. Embarrassment, shame, and anger welled up inside me. Desperate, I ordered Alexa to watch Caleb while I dragged my rag doll through the parking lot. Joshy was going big guns for this tantrum, evidenced by his attempt at the wet noodle. He lay limp on the pavement, screaming his head off, while he thrashed and flailed his limbs. I was kicked and punched repeatedly. My strong-willed child refused to move. The only way Joshy would have gotten into the van was if a tornado swept him up and carried him there.

At first I didn't speak much because I feared Joshy was craving negative attention from me. But honestly, I didn't have anything kind or coherent to say, and I didn't have a clue what I was doing. I attempted to strap him into his car seat but my efforts proved futile against his strength provided by the powerful adrenaline coursing through his veins. Joshy and I both were unsafe to drive or ride in the van until we calmed down. I found myself screaming and crying right along with him, insisting he stop.

By now the other kids were crying and covering their ears, too. Out of anger and desperation, I finally grabbed Joshy by the arm and roughly yanked him outside the van. I refused to let him back in until he calmed down. He punched the windows and kicked the side panel, but I still did not let him back in. To this day I still cannot *believe I actually locked my three-year-old son out of the van*. It makes my stomach turn just thinking how cruel I must have been. My only defense is that I was suffering, scared, and crazed in that moment. Thankfully, it only took me a few minutes to see that my efforts were futile. Resigned, I walked around to sit by Joshy on the hot asphalt where I cradled him in my lap until he was done sobbing thirty minutes later. He couldn't even remember why he became upset in the first place.

The tantrums with Joshy were many, but the Lord taught me a critical lesson through it all. Never ever, ever, ever judge another parent or child who is misbehaving in a public place. Prior to my own experiences, I was the judge and accuser. Whenever my peaceful trip to the store was interrupted by a screaming, flailing child I would label their parents as spineless, inconsistent, or clueless.

Now I was able to internalize scripture, "Why do you look at the speck of sawdust in your brother's eye and pay no attention to the plank in your own eye?" (Matthew 7:3) God was certainly teaching me through very harsh circumstances. You just never know what struggles that family endures. I have walked their shoes and felt their pain.

PRAYER WARRIORS

While we lived in Warsaw, we attended the Wesleyan Church. Christi introduced me to her circle of friends, and I immediately plugged myself into a charismatic prayer group. Oh how I miss those nights of fervent prayer! One evening when we started to pray, somebody felt led by the Spirit to read Psalm 32. Verses 4-5 resonated in my soul:

> When I kept silent, my bones wasted away through my groaning all day long. For day and night your hand was heavy upon me; my strength was sapped as in the heat of the summer. Then I acknowledged my sin to you and did not cover up my iniquity. I said 'I will confess my sin to you and you did not cover up my iniquity.' I said, 'I will confess my transgressions to the Lord' *and you forgave me the guilt of my sin.*

The hairs bristled all over my body and I started to shiver. Saltwater droplets streamed down my rosy cheeks. In that moment I realized I was being convicted by the Holy Spirit of my sin and guilt over my recent behavior toward my son. The weight upon my shoulders felt like an anvil smashing me down; it was as if I my mind and body were suffocating from the burden. I took a quick glance upward to see if my girlfriends were all staring at me. Maybe I had a large *s* on my forehead showcasing me with the "All-Time Sinner Award." Yet the girls were still praying, eyes down. Don't my girlfriends know that this is a rebuke to me from the Father? The passage was also encouragement, yet in that moment I was completely blinded by my own shame. The guilt of my imperfectness nearly crippled me.

As the passage closed, I could no longer contain the raw emotion within. Convicted of my behavior toward my son and marveling that the Lord chose to speak to *me* that night, I purged all of my regrets, fears, and perceived inadequacies with my sisters in Christ. Until this moment I carried such a heavy burden for this child I loved more than life itself. That night I was finally able to experience relief from the oppression by sharing with the group how seriously my son was struggling and how desperate I was to find answers and relief. They lifted me up in intercessory prayer and spoke like angels on my behalf. Free at last. The guilt, regret, sorrow, and grief melted away as the rusty shackles that bound my hands and feet were released.

Joshy was lifted up in prayer a million times thereafter because I had a team of faithful prayer warriors that believed in God's divine intervention. And I still break down on my knees, weeping and asking for forgiveness for all the terrible times I yelled and lost patience. I was also reminded by a good friend of God's promise in Psalm 103:12. "As far as the east is from the west, so far has he removed our transgressions from us." Glory be to God! *You mean all the horrible thoughts I have, all the terrible moments of yelling are just…gone? You mean you promise me that all my baggage goes into the wilderness of forgetfulness? How could I be so lucky, Lord?*

THE VINE

I t was difficult to determine if Joshy's emotional outbursts were intentional. Once I made the grave mistake of making it a control issue when it was not. I just couldn't let him win. I reasoned, *if I give in and simply console him, does that mean Joshy wins? Or do I need to stay strong and stick to the consequences so he learns?* On the one hand, I knew Joshy had been diagnosed with a mood disorder, but on the other hand, his behavior was simply inexcusable. I just couldn't let him win the fights. It took me many more incidents over the next couple of years to realize that no, Joshy was never winning. There was no delight in this power struggle, only fear and suffering.

My confusion made it difficult to delineate what was typical childhood development for a boy versus what was part of an emotional disability? Compounding my dilemma was that Joshy was a very big boy, so there became a massive discrepancy between his chronological age and his maturity and behavior. Dave's height is a whopping six feet six inches, so I know where Joshy's size comes from. When he was three-years-old, he had the body of a five-year-old yet the mind of a toddler, making it nearly impossible to come up with consistent, age appropriate expectations.

This discrepancy was apparent when we placed Joshy in a private preschool at the age of three. By developmental standards he should have entered the program with fine motor and communication skills like the other three year olds. But to the teachers his tall, lanky body and bright inquisitive eyes were met with expectations of a boy the age of five. Naturally they were stunned when he could not speak clearly or write a few lowercase letters in the alphabet.

I secretly observed Joshy in the classroom through many hallway windows. I was also privy to the side glances the teachers made to each other when they were unsuccessful at helping him. Perhaps the most striking deficit I witnessed was Joshy's social/emotional delays. Although he craved attention and interaction with the children he simply did not understand how to play with them. He engaged in parallel play rather than reciprocal play and he struggled with turn taking and sharing. Joshy was easily frustrated with simple demands which resulted in exaggerated screaming fits conducted by a toddler. He that could not figure out how to communicate his needs appropriately.

Finally the teachers confided to me their concerns. They admitted that there were evident delays, and these delays seemed to be much worse than original expectations because they were comparing him to a *five year old based on his size and stature*. It just didn't seem fair.

I begged God to be softer with his teachings and not allow these life lessons to hurt so much, but He knew I needed the sting of the experience or my heart would never change. I started feeling like the pruned vine to which Jesus refers in John 15: 1-2 (ESV):

> I a.m. the True Vine, and My Father is the Vinedresser. Any branch in Me that does not bear fruit He cuts away; and He cleanses and repeatedly prunes every branch that continues to bear fruit, to make it bear more and richer and more excellent fruit.

Maybe my branch produced only rotten fruit, and that was why the Lord gave me such an extensive pruning. I'm still not sure. I hoped that my pruning season was complete so that I would be free to produce an abundance of good, healthy fruit. Plus, this pruning hurt!

A PARENT'S GRIEF

The Old Testament story of Hagar and Ishmael, described in Genesis 16 and 21 has always been close to my heart. The story begins with Abraham and Sarah unable to conceive a child. Desperate, Sarah convinced Abraham to sleep with her maidservant Hagar, and they conceived a boy named Ishmael. But Sarah's ingenious plan backfired; she seethed with jealousy while Abraham and Hagar bonded during the pregnancy. Sarah's bitterness ran deep.

When Hagar could bear no more abuse from Sarah, she ran away from the torment to hide and protect her unborn child, but an angel of the Lord instructed her to return. The angel of the lord prophesized to Hagar about her son Ishmael:

> This son of yours will be a wild man, as untamed as a wild donkey! He will raise his fist against everyone, and everyone will be against him. Yes, he will live in open hostility against all his relatives.
>
> Genesis 16:12 (NLT)

Not the best welcoming for a newborn about to enter this world. Hagar reluctantly but obediently returned.

Genesis 17:16 describes how Ishmael grew up. When his father, Abraham, and Sarah became very old, the Lord miraculously blessed them with their very own son, who they named Isaac. A ninety-year-old woman and one-hundred-year-old man were promised to conceive a child! The imminent birth of Isaac stirred up tension again between the two mothers, Sarah and Hagar. Sadly, Abraham sent Hagar and Ishmael away to keep peace at the home front. Rejected and scared, mother and son wandered aimlessly into the desert. Genesis 21:14-21 describes Hagar's despair:

> Hagar went on her way and wandered in the desert of Beersheba. When the water in the skin was gone, she put the boy under one of the bushes. Then she went off and sat down nearby, about a bowshot away, for she thought, "I cannot watch the boy die." And as she sat there nearby, she began to sob. God heard the boy crying, and the angel of God called to Hagar from heaven and said to her, "What is the matter, Hagar? Do not be afraid; God has heard the boy crying as he lies there. Lift the boy up and take him by the hand, for I will make him into a great nation." Then God opened her eyes and she saw a well of water. So she went and filled the skin with water and gave the boy a drink. God was with the boy as he grew up. He lived in the desert and became an archer.

I have poured over this story many nights relating to what Hagar must have experienced. *She left her son under a bush to die and walked away.* Why? Hagar simply could not bear to see him die. She could not watch him suffer through life, endure pain, or face death.

The Lord did something else for Hagar and Ishmael that was amazing. He allowed his very own heart to break at the sight of this mother and son confronting such a frightening future. *As the mother sobbed, God unleashed his loving kindness.* He refreshed and restored both of them with water and hope. The Lord felt the same pain for Hagar that she felt for Ishmael, and that I felt for my son. *Thank you, Lord for Your compassion and empathy that surrounds us!*

It is easy as parents to empathize with Hagar's pain because The Lord has created us with such depth of emotion for our children. Tragedies such as the loss of a child or a child's disability are heinous to endure. While I have felt like Hagar many times, this passage helps me realize that my heartbreak for my son was not the first or the last heartbreak in eternity. I am not alone in my grief.

It took me awhile to surrender to my grief. At first I thought my grief was so selfish, so I kept my feelings of bitterness hidden in my heart. I did not want to address it anyway, it was too painful. But slowly I started to realize that even if I didn't talk about the grief, my feelings remained. Besides, the Lord knew my thoughts and fears anyway. It just took time, confession, and a lot of honesty.

I grieved over a lost childhood for Joshua. I grieved over my fractured family and the shattered visions of happy family vacations and summer breaks. And I grieved over the tenuous relationships Joshua had with each member in our family. I grieved that my life as a mother was not as I expected. After I finally surrendered and released my heartache, I experienced a freedom I never had before.

As I remembered Hagar and Ishmael I knew I was not alone. I was also comforted knowing that the Lord understood how I felt because He allowed his precious son Jesus to suffer and die for me. The Lord didn't stop his flesh and blood from dying an excruciating, humiliating death although he could have because He is Lord! Instead God's heart crumbled watching His son suffer on Calvary.

Finally, Hagar and Ishmael's story fills me with *hope*. The Lord encouraged Hagar to remain with her son and *never give up*. He promised to lift Ishmael up and make him a great nation. There was hope for Ishmael; there is hope for Joshua.

HE'S MY SON

As Joshy and I struggled to navigate our relationship each day, I turned back to what was familiar and comforting—music. But to say I *turned* to music is an understatement; I actually *immersed* myself in music. I completely engrossed myself in worship all day and night. You could guarantee music was playing throughout my house or car twenty-four-seven. Dave and I purchased an electronic keyboard with microphones so we could praise Jesus together in the evening. Joshy and Alexa would both take turns singing "Open the Eyes of My Heart Lord" (Michael W. Smith, 2001) with voices of a thousand angels. Singing continues to be my healing rain; it washes over me, comforts me, and draws me closer to God.

Mark Shultz is Christian artist and gifted songwriter, musician, and storyteller whose lyrics have always touched my heart. I especially cherished one song released around this time, entitled "He's My Son" (Mark Shultz, 2000). I bought the track and memorized every lyric, feeling certain the Lord was speaking to me and that this was to become my own personal prayer:

> Can You hear me? Am I getting through tonight?
> See, he's not just anyone, he's my son.

Seven years later the Lord took take my hand and granted me the privilege of singing this powerful, poignant, very personal song for my congregation. The Lord lifted me up as I allowed myself to be exposed, vulnerable, and real. This was my way of healing.

THE WHISPER OF GOD

In addition to worship, I also began searching for more guidance and perspective through a stringent schedule of meditation and prayer. I spent countless afternoons pleading for God to speak to me, when finally, one afternoon, I heard His whisper. I can only describe it as a gentle voice wafting into my soul, as if it was carried by a breeze coming in the window. It was a breeze that I could feel *inside*. My typical senses were of no use. I couldn't see or hear, but I felt His presence.

My pen and paper flowed freely on the Post-It note in front of me; it was as if my hand was not my own to control:

> Do you trust me Jamie? *Yes I do, Lord.* Do you know that my way is perfect because I love you? *Yes Lord, I also know this.* Do you also know that I love your son even more than you do? *Yes Lord, I must leave him to you. He is your child.* Rest in me, Jamie. Rest in Me for every hurt. I will never let you fall. *Oh Father, please help my son. Help him only as you can, and let me be as loving and patient with him as you are with me.*

I've kept this Post-It note safe in a box to share with Joshy someday, so he can see all the amazing ways the Lord has touched our lives.

PART 2

THE WILDERNESS

Although we loved Warsaw and would have been content to live there forever, Dave's company, owned by Johnson & Johnson, had been trying for months to convince him to accept a promotion based out of their corporate headquarters near Piscataway, New Jersey. For many months we procrastinated on the decision, but it was becoming time for Dave to advance his career. When we finally made the heart wrenching decision to leave Warsaw, I was scared to death. I clung to what Scripture promises in Deuteronomy 31:6, "Be strong! Be courageous! Do not be afraid of them! For the Lord your God will be with you. He will neither fail you nor forsake you."

In April 2004, after four goodbye parties, we packed our bags and headed east. Although I was excited to move across the country, I was crestfallen at the prospect of being separated from my church, family, Christi, and Mary and Chad. With promises to everybody that distance only makes hearts grow fonder, we left our spiritual pillars of strength. Our life was suddenly catapulted to Easton, Pennsylvania, sardonically termed the desert.

I thought I could handle Pennsylvania despite my losses back in Indiana because I knew in my heart I was never alone. After all, God promised me in Joshua 1:5-9 (NASB):

> Be strong and courageous, for you shall give this people possession of the land which I swore to their fathers to give them. Only be strong and very courageous; be careful to do according to all the law which Moses My servant commanded you; do not turn from it to the right or to the left, so that you may have success wherever you go. This book of the law shall not depart from your mouth,

but you shall meditate on it day and night, so that you may be careful to do according to all that is written in it; for then you will make your way prosperous, and then you will have success. Have I not commanded you? Be strong and courageous! Do not tremble or be dismayed, for the LORD your God is with you wherever you go.

This verse carried me through the transition into our new world. I knew I had to stay close to the Word and keep my relationship with the Lord a priority. He made it clear through his Word and circumstances that I needed to be strong and courageous, so I tried my best to give my fears over to Him on those lonely, somber nights.

Dr. H

Before we moved to Easton, Joshy was already taking an increased dose of Risperdal because his body built up a tolerance over time to the smaller amount. This is a typical phenomenon, but I found it disconcerting that my forty pound child needed higher dosages of antipsychotic drugs. Joshy continued to have explosive mood swings, so Depakote (an anti-convulsant mediation) was also added into his daily regime. I was skeptical that the Depakote was helping because extreme impulsivity and hyperactivity continued on a daily basis. Dave and I agreed to attempt the non-stimulant medication Straterra, but that was ineffective at decreasing his ADHD symptoms. Reluctantly, we also tried the stimulant Concerta, yet this only agitated him. It sickened me that my son was essentially a guinea pig for all these mediation trials. I finally gave up on there ever being a remedy for his ADHD symptoms.

When we were settled into our new home, my first priority was to start searching for a new psychiatrist. I only had two choices within a fifty mile radius because nobody would treat Joshy with a ten foot pole because he was only the tender age of four. Twenty phone calls and a few phone interviews later, I settled on psychiatrist Dr. Hammond (Dr. H). The hour commute to his office was a small sacrifice if it meant he could help my son. Dr. H was a foreign, elderly gentleman with a great passion for treating pediatric mental illness. Unfortunately, his thick accent made it difficult for any of us to communicate with him, and he really was quite old; I worried that he might not be on top of the latest research and medication available.

Every appointment was torture for me and the kids. If they weren't confined on the car ride, they certainly were limited in his tiny office. There were only a few toys to play with, and Joshy usually destroyed them while engaging in screaming wars with his brother and sister. It was electrified sensory overload for even the experienced psychiatrist. Dr. H confirmed Joshy's diagnoses as ADHD and Bipolar Disorder. He also diagnosed Joshy with a Phonological Processing Disorder, as Joshy's articulation was clearly delayed; it was becoming increasingly difficult to understand him.

Dr. H continued Joshy's treatment with Risperdal and Concerta, but he changed the Depakote to Topamax. Topamax was another anti-convulsant medication, typically prescribed to prevent seizures and migraine headaches by decreasing abnormal excitement in the brain. Research had shown that it could also be successful in regulating moods (Topomax, 2011). We gave it the good old college try, but we had to discontinue the Topomax after two weeks. Unfortunately Joshy could not tolerate it due to extreme fatigue, decreased appetite, and weight loss.

EARLY INTERVENTION

When I searched for assistance and services for Joshy, I discovered an early intervention program in Bethlehem called Colonial Intermediate Unit 20. I scheduled an intake assessment right away, and this time the results indicated multiple areas of developmental delays. At the age of four years and two months, Joshy's skills were only that of a two- or three-year-old boy. *What could have possibly happened to make his development slow down, Lord? This makes no sense!*

Since significant delays were established across all areas, Joshy qualified for early intervention services through the public preschools. A team of special education teachers and therapists crafted an individualized education plan and invited Joshy to their program. He worked with a special education teacher, speech therapist, and occupational therapist. Together they started to work on fine motor skills, social kills, and behavior management.

Each week Joshy rode the big yellow bus to school. He was positively determined to embark upon his educational journey! My little boy had to work twenty times harder to accomplish so many things we all take for granted, but he never gave up. Every day I eagerly awaited the bus coming over the distant horizon. Usually I would find him exhausted and asleep in his car seat with "blankie" resting on his cheek. Such a hard day's work for a sweet, little soul. All of the attention and therapy sparked Joshy to make slow but steady gains.

The social skills class also helped develop his God-given gift of empathy. While it was easy for Joshy to internalize empathy, most children with significant social deficits find it extremely difficult to understand another person's feelings. But Joshy could always recognize another's need for help and give assistance, and if he sensed sadness within another's soul, he would cry right along with them. My heart swelled and melted when I saw his empathy toward others. I often caught him consoling his baby brother or friends in the neighborhood with candy or hugs and kisses.

There may have been a war raging inside Joshy's head, but there was a gentle soul within. Joshy became extremely affectionate with everyone; he could never snuggle close enough and always needed to be holding my hand. He was extraordinarily sensitive to other's emotional states. He was the boy with the box of Kleenex at the movie. When we saw *Marley & Me* (2005) at the movie theatre, he sobbed until there were no tears left.

Joshy made his first attempt at group sports that fall; he made such an adorable soccer goalie. His first great feat was winning the ball and then kicking it into his *own* goal. He was so proud of himself, smiling and waving to the crowd, he had all the parents cheering. Although he loved soccer, it was short lived. When he was on the field, his brain could not process the action and strategy quickly enough. Joshy would just stand there, frozen, not knowing where to turn. His foot rarely touched the ball. The chaos of the game, the strategy, and the foot skills required were not meshing with his strengths at that time, and he became easily frustrated. We decided to look for something else when the time was right.

MEDICAL MYSTERY NUMBER 2

Joshy missed his grandparents terribly, so he was delighted when he learned both sides of the family were coming for a visit for Caleb's first birthday in October. Celebrating and reconnecting with family was magnificent. Joshy even had two consistent days of emotional stability. But by the third morning of my family's visit, Joshy awoke crying out in great pain when he tried to get out of bed. He had an intermittent fever, which we treated with Tylenol, but otherwise, his listless body just lied on the floor, clearly uncomfortable in his own skin.

By the next morning, Joshy still couldn't bear weight without crumbling into a heap. I was becoming anxious to make a decision on where to take him. *Do we ride this out like before? Or do we take what little money we have and trust in the doctor?* I was reassured by Proverbs 3:5-8:

> Trust in the Lord with all your heart and lean not on your own understanding. In all your ways acknowledge Him, and He will make your paths straight. Do not be wise in your own eyes; fear the Lord and shun evil. This will bring health to your body and nourishment to your bones.

How can I argue with that Lord? Off to the hospital we go. We chose the Emergency Room at St. Luke's Hospital in Bethlehem. We tried to get Joshy to indicate the area of greatest pain, but he could only place his hands upon his upper thighs and hips with a whimper. X-rays and CT Scans revealed normal findings. Blood tests revealed high white blood cell counts and a low lymphocyte count again, similar to what we found at Lutheran Hospital two years prior.

One test indicated a positive ASO Titer for Strepptococcus which suggested Joshy may have recently been exposed to strep throat that went untreated. *He never complained of a sore throat! Poor baby!* I supposed it wasn't surprising that he never told me his throat hurt because he struggled to communicate even the most basic needs such as pain or hunger at times. A Lyme Total Antibody Screen was also performed, which turned out negative. However, there was a disclaimer attached in his personal records that read, "Positive results may be delayed for up to 8 weeks after onset of illness. Antibiotic therapy may lead to false negative results." *Hmm…Joshy has been on and off antibiotics for many months due to constant upper respiratory infections.*

Perplexed, the doctors admitted Joshy into the hospital for observation. Dave and I split our time at the hospital, and after he would fall asleep in the evening, we would go home for a short nap. Meanwhile, each day I was getting more frustrated with the staff because it seemed like they weren't doing any investigating or collaborating about what might ail Joshy while he grew more restless in his pale, sterile room.

When I visited Joshy, he was temperamental with me and the nurses. My only motive was to come in to snuggle and comfort my baby, but this four-year-old tyrant was making that quite difficult. As Joshy started regaining his ability to walk again, he would scream at me and tear off down the corridors. He was uncontrollable and refused to listen to any limitation placed upon him. He was psychologically and physically miserable inside and out. It got to the point that as much as I couldn't wait to visit him, *I didn't want to visit him.* I was riddled with guilt for feeling this way.

After three days in the hospital, Joshy was finally discharged because the symptoms spontaneously abated. Their diagnosis was "rheumatic fever" since he had strep throat that went untreated. Reluctantly we returned home.

Back at home we kept Joshy's physical activity to a minimum, but within two more days Joshy could not walk again! The symptoms were so surreal that we started wondering if he was making this up for attention. Since I was jaded by my experience at St. Luke's, I decided we must travel to a well respected Children's hospital for quality medical care. With all three kids in tow, Dave and I headed down to Children's Hospital of Philadelphia (CHOP). After a two hour drive and a three hour wait in the emergency room, we finally were able to present our case to a team of emergency doctors.

The doctors conducted an abbreviated physical exam and read the discharge papers from St. Luke's. Within ten measly minutes they assuredly claimed, "Joshua has tenosynovitis in his hips." *He has what?* They patiently described the problem, "Tenosynovitis is when inflammation and fluid build up in the sheath surrounding tendons, and in your son's case, it's the tendons surrounding his joints in his hips. This can manifest as pain and difficulty moving the particular joints where the inflammation occurs." He was sent home with instructions to take Ibuprofen and rest. *Wow, tenosynovitis is a far cry from rheumatic fever. What is really going on, Lord?*

JESUS TAKE THE WHEEL

We wanted to introduce a personalized sport for Joshy to help him work out some of his extra energy and encourage positive social skills, so karate seemed like a fabulous match. It was touted to increase self esteem, attention, and self control. Unfortunately, after three sessions, Joshy was still clinging to my legs, pleading with me not to leave. Unfortunately, his fear of leaving me was still too great at this stage for him to be successful with any sport.

Although the karate was a bust, the car ride to karate class one evening forever changed his life. One evening Joshy started asking me spiritual questions regarding Papa John's death. Joshy was extremely close to his step grandfather when he lost a valiant but short battle to lung cancer last fall. I felt so terrible that Joshy did not have the expressive language skills to articulate his concerns six months earlier.

"Mommy, where did Papa John go?"

"Sweetie, Papa John's soul went to heaven, but his shell was left behind."

With tears forming, Joshy confided, "I have been sad and scared since then because I thought we just left him all alone in the box at the funeral home in the dark."

Joshy was very literal, so it was no wonder he assumed this. This was a perfect opportunity to explain to Joshy that Papa John was very much not alone because he went to heaven to dance with the angels. I explained that our shell stays behind on earth, but our hearts and souls float up to heaven.

"How do you know, Mommy?"

"Because Papa John had a personal relationship with the Lord."

"What does that mean, Mommy?"

I tried to explain, "Well, do you remember last month when you drew crayon over the walls even though you knew it was wrong? We all do bad things even though we want to be good. And we keep trying to be good, but we keep doing bad things, even Mommy and Daddy! These bad things sometimes keep us far away from God. But there is a way to keep him close forever and ever...."

Joshy interjected, "What do you mean, Mommy?"

"Well, the Bible says in Romans 10:9-10, 'If you confess with your mouth, "Jesus is Lord," and believe in your heart that God raised him from the dead, you will be saved. For it is with your heart that you believe and are justified, and it is with your mouth that you confess and are saved.'"

"What does *that* mean, Mommy?"

"It means all you have to do is say a special prayer so that someday you can go to heaven to live with Jesus and Papa John forever!"

Eyes beaming, Joshy said, "Yes, Mommy! Let's do it!"

I pulled the car over to the side of the road, joy rushing into my heart. Joshy repeated after me a simple, beautiful prayer that ended with him asking Jesus to come into his life and live in his heart. We were both crying, knowing that Joshy's heart was cleansed through Jesus. We placed a white rose on the altar at church that Sunday in celebration of his decision.

But Satan did not like this one bit. He was most definitely thinking, "How dare Joshy get closer to the kingdom of God!" Satan fought against anything positive in Joshy's life. He was always plotting, always putting obstacles and limitations across Joshy's path. Yet my confidence was strong that the Almighty One was truly in control.

THE ABYSS

I continued my attempts to discover alternative treatment options for Joshy. I signed him up for a music therapy class to help his social skills. I took all dyes out of his diet because I had heard that could cause hyperactivity or irritability. I even purchased the probiotic acidophilus to help his immune and digestive system. But nothing worked! I was pulling my hair out from frustration! Despite my faith and my best attempts at a well-balanced life, I still believed I was failing miserably.

My own self-deprecating thoughts gave birth to self-hatred. I felt so hideous inside. I had taken the antidepressant Prozac when I developed post partum depression after my first pregnancy, but it was not enough to carry me through this abyss. I started to become paranoid that perhaps I had a mood disorder as well. *Could I have passed it on to my son?* My thoughts raced all the time, I had insomnia, and I would vacillate between tears and laughter frequently.

I finally made my own private appointment with Dr. H. to see if he could help me as well. Dr. H helped me distinguish between depression with anxiety, and a mood disorder. He asked me if I liked the way it felt when my thoughts were racing or I was not sleeping.

"No! Of course I don't like it. I hate it! It's such an uncomfortable sensation; I just want to stop thinking about my problems so much!"

Dr. H explained to me that it was unlikely I had a mood disorder. When somebody is truly manic, the euphoria they feel is wonderful and all encompassing. They never want it to end. But when somebody has racing thoughts, worry, and sadness and it makes them feel miserable, that is not likely a mood imbalance. He felt certain that my highly stressful situation was causing anxiety and depression. I was grateful he helped me distinguish between the two so that was one less thing to worry about.

The negative side to my visit with Dr. H. is that he stopped my long term, "steady Eddie" antidepressant Prozac and prescribed Topamax instead to help with my own mood fluctuations. I'm not sure why he did that considering he was the one who specifically stated I did not have a mood disorder. Nevertheless, I was initially excited to try this medication because I had listened to a close friend's testimony about the efficacy of this medicine, Topamax was also known to help with weight loss—added bonus! I had to slowly titrate up the dosage the first few weeks to reach a therapeutic dosage.

Trying Topamax became a disaster. The first problem I encountered was constant tingling and numbness down my arms; it was quite bothersome as it would not go away. The second problem was that I was becoming a zombie without realizing it. The medication simply took me out of this world. After I started the Topamax, Dave and I took the eight hour journey out to Ohio with the kids, and I was literally an incoherent blob for the entire ride. I couldn't muster the energy to interact with the children, and I slept for hours at a time. Dave was alarmed by my sedation, but the drug prevented me from being able to look outside myself and see what was really happening. Each day I woke up and found myself in a place I didn't even recognize anymore. I was a thirty-something mother and wife who literally could not put one foot in front of the other to start my day. My day only meant hardship and misery, and parenting seemed to be a thankless, miserable job. I couldn't make my boy happy. I couldn't force him to have self-control. I couldn't ease his pain.

I would look in my bathroom mirror at my reflection and not recognize the woman staring back at me. Late each night after everybody went to sleep, I would take a dangerous sleeping pill and crawl into my jet-tub bath. I would soak for hours, drifting in and out of consciousness while sinking down deeper and deeper into the water. I often fell asleep until my head went under water; only then would life be shaken back into me.

I admitted to myself that I wanted to die; I had no reason to go on. I started to believe that Satan won, and that Joshy's life would only be full of trials and discontentment. My work was done, and I failed. It would never get any better. This was the darkest period of my life and it gives me the shivers to revisit these emotions. Words cannot express the depth of the despair and hopelessness I experienced. I felt doomed to carry this burden my entire life! I hated God and cursed the day He gave me life. I couldn't face my insecurities as a parent and couldn't deal with another day of not knowing how to help my son.

I shudder to recall the dread that swept over me every morning as I approached the entryway into Joshy's bedroom. I knew that as soon as I crossed its threshold, we would begin another ten continuous hours of struggles. Yet right when I would feel I could not sink any lower, a letter would arrive from Christi:

> Jamie, remember that Matthew 11:28 says "Come to me all you who are heavy leaden and I will give you rest." This promise covers the excess questioning and self-doubt and self-guilt that we as humans place upon ourselves as a pseudo-replacement for our inability to make sense of things. We only cloud the moment when we question "why" continually.

God always sent her to me at the perfect moment. In my drug-induced haze, this verse gave me the encouragement I needed to finally reach out to my sister Jessica and confide that I was having suicidal thoughts. She was an amazing counselor and suggested that for starters I get off this darned Topamax. She called me diligently and spoke my love language by sending me meaningful music. Within a few days of ceasing the Topamax, I restarted my old antidepressant. Immediately the fog cleared from my mind and I was able to look at the past month with a fresh, clear perspective. I was in absolute shock over what transpired and how close I came to the edge of despair.

Slowly, I started to confide in a few friends about my suicidal thoughts and how I had never before felt despair like this in my entire life. No matter how disappointed or desperate I felt, I always believed God was in control and there was a rainbow around every corner until this abyss. After sharing my vulnerability, I was stunned to hear every single one of them admit they had felt the exact same way not once, but multiple times in their lives. I couldn't understand how they treated the idea of suicide so nonchalantly! My friends almost seemed to accept that it was a rite of passage everybody goes through. At least I wasn't alone.

I did a little research on Topamax and found many instances where the drug induced suicidal ideation in otherwise mentally healthy individuals. *Unbelievable.* I wanted to sue the manufacturers, but I knew I didn't have enough energy or money to deal with a lawsuit. Instead, I focused on positive things. I read excerpts from *The Father's Love Letter* constantly. I treasured these words and verses from Scripture that I believed my Father was speaking to me and Joshy:

> …. For I am your greatest encourager. I am also the Father who comforts you… My child, you may not know me, but I know everything about you. I know when you sit down and when you rise up. I am familiar with all your

ways. Even the very hairs on your head are numbered. For you were made in my image. In me you live and move and have your being. For you are my offspring. I knew you even before you were conceived. I chose you when I planned creation. You were not a mistake, for all your days are written in my book. I determined the exact time of your birth and where you would live. You are fearfully and wonderfully made. I knit you together in your mother's womb…. And it is my desire to lavish my love on you. Simply because you are my child and I am your Father…. My plan for your future has always been filled with hope. Because I love you with an everlasting love. My thoughts toward you are countless as the sand on the seashore. And I rejoice over you with singing. When you are brokenhearted, I am close to you. As a shepherd carries a lamb, I have carried you close to my heart. One day I will wipe away every tear from your eyes. And I'll take away all the pain you have suffered on this earth. I am your Father, and I love you even as I love my son, Jesus.

Waves of comfort would wash over me with these words from the Scriptures. It provided such an affirmation that in our uniqueness Joshy and I were loved by our father and creator. I felt covered, as if I could fall into the arms of this brilliant craftsman and protector. But most of all, in the midst of chaos I felt God's promise for our futures and our life everlasting. Every day I wrestle at the enormity of His love despite my imperfections.

SPIRITUAL WARFARE

During the spring of 2004, we registered Joshy at the House of Rock Christian Preschool for the days he was not attending the early intervention program. In this setting Joshy did not have a personal classroom aide, which meant that completion of pre-readiness activities and navigating social relationships were difficult. I would get reports each week that Joshy did not respect other's personal space and that he had hit some boy or pulled some girl's hair.

We were also increasingly concerned with his expressive speech and articulation. Not only did he struggle to express himself, but when he tried, his words were muffled and slurred together. I started to worry that the other children would notice Joshy was different and not want to be friends with him...it was a cruel world out there, after all. Whenever these insecurities flooded my heart, I was reminded that my fear was based on my lack of trust in the Lord's ability to protect Joshy. I had to pray for blind faith and trust in Him every single day to combat my fears.

Striving to be a proactive parent and help Joshy with his speech skills, I found a great audio CD that enabled children to isolate speech sounds and practice them repetitively. Unfortunately, my solution morphed into a cataclysmic nightmare. One morning I introduced the CD to Joshy while we were driving to preschool. I was happily trying the speech sounds to encourage him while I drove the car. After the CD played for about two minutes Joshy became agitated and started screaming "Stop! Stop the voices!"

I had just arrived at the church, so I slammed on the brakes in the parking lot and ran around to open his side door. The CD was no longer playing, but he continued to cry and chant, "Please stop the voices!" I held my hands tightly against his pudgy cheeks and asked him what he was hearing. Crying, in incomplete and incoherent sentences, I pieced together that there were voices taunting him, hissing "Joshua, Joshua." Waves of chills ran down my spine and my blood ran cold. Goosebumps rippled up the flesh of my arms and my brain started whirling with clarity. Adrenaline kicked in as strongly as my spiritual discernment. There were only two things I knew in that moment:

1. (one) This was not a joke
2. (two) This was *not* of God.

Later that night I had an epiphany: Easton, Pennsylvania was Joshy's desert as it was mine. Throughout this barren, desolate wilderness in which the Lord placed us, I realized it was not enough to only accept the Lord's sovereignty over our lives. Just as critical, we had to acknowledge the evil one's plans to separate us from the Almighty One.

Joshy's struggles challenged me to ask the question regarding what was so ominous about Satan. I found my answer in a passage in Job 1: 6-7. In this chapter, when both the angels and Satan approached the Lord, the Lord asked Satan, "Where have you come from?" Satan answered, "From roaming through the earth and going back and forth in it." I realized that Satan is depicted as an *active adversary*—trolling our world, seeking out ways to destroy us. Despite Satan's attempts to make life difficult I was determined not to live in fear. God and His goodness are always most powerful. Demons are described in the commentary notes of the NIV Bible as "fallen angels who joined Satan in his rebellion against God and are now evil spirits under Satan's control. They help Satan tempt people to sin and have great destructive powers." But listen closely to what it says next. *"But whenever they are confronted by Jesus, they lose their power."* I surmised that Satan was not making this journey easy, but ultimately the Lord was in control and would be the victor!

Meanwhile, Joshy continued to be tormented by the hissing, haunting voices. Although the voices never gave him directives, they did cause continual chaos and fear in his mind. Since I knew that my God was not a God of chaos, but of peace and order, I realized that Joshy was particularly susceptible and vulnerable to spiritual warfare. Suddenly my worldly standards collided with my spiritual beliefs. I became conflicted between my old counseling theories and my newly heightened awareness of spiritual warfare. Scripture most certainly says spiritual warfare exists, yet many choose to ignore this because the concept seems unfamiliar, scary, and downright unpleasant. I also knew from the top of my head to the tips of my toes that these voices were not part of a mental illness. Instead, there was something *not of God* within him—he was possessed by an evil spirit or demon. This epiphany was way bigger than me. *Why him, Lord? Why me? I am a weak, fallible, mere human! You cannot possibly expect me to fight off the evil one on his behalf!*

AN EXCELLENT WAY

I started looking for answers and clinging to hope through my research on healing ministries. Eventually I settled upon a trans-denominational ministry led by Pastor Henry Wright at Pleasant Valley Church in Thomaston, Georgia. I purchased Wright's esteemed book, *A More Excellent Way* (Dr. Henry Wright, 2005). I devoured his writing and my discernment found his words to be biblically sound.

Wright is committed to his theory that human problems are fundamentally spiritual, with associated physical and psychological manifestations. He also believes that the root of psychological and biological disease is spiritual. His book explained the biblical basis for why mankind has disease, the spiritual roots of disease, and blocks to healing. Wright offers solutions for his primary goal of disease prevention and eradication. I could relate to this ministry and it appeared authentic.

I wasn't convinced with all of Wright's theories regarding the root causes of specific diseases, but his lesson on generational curses certainly hit home. I reflected upon the lives of my father and my father's father, and I saw some very specific weaknesses and sinful tendencies passed down the family line manifesting within myself. Generational curses are insidious. They quietly creep inside and take over your heart, despite your adamant desire to do things differently than your parents. I humbly took ownership of a prayer that Dr. Wright provided (2005):

> In the name of Jesus, in the power of His Blood, and in the full and finished work of the Cross, I now rebuke, break and loose, myself and my family from any and all evil curses that have been put upon us through our own

sins or the sins of our ancestors. Break the power of and dissolve every curse, bond, dedication, spiritual chain or spiritual influence over me and over my family.

Father God in Jesus' name, I confess and freely forgive all my ancestors for all sins and weaknesses which may have affected me and my family and hereby forgive and bless those persons through whom the curses came. I ask you to forgive and bless them as well. I also ask You to forgive me for any curses I have put on others through the wrong use of my tongue. I renounce my own evil words and pray for the liberation of those whom I have injured.

Father, I now ask you in Jesus name, and by His full and finished work, to take back the ground that was given up to the enemy through any involvement with him. I ask you, Lord, that the door be closed and sealed with Your precious Blood. From this day forward I will walk in Your blessings and live in obedience. Amen!

This prayer became an essential part of my armor that shielded me from the evil one while I continued my journey to find healing for my son.

GEORGIA

D ave supported my investigation into spiritual healing because he loved us, he believed in the power of Christ, and he knew I did not want to live with regret or have any stone left unturned. Consequently, he purchased me two tickets to Georgia to Dr. Wright's healing ministry for the following week.

Although I was fueled with adrenalin and optimism about this journey, I was reticent with most people. I was even scared to tell my family where I was going for fear they would think I was too radical. One of my biggest weaknesses has always been esteeming what others thought of me above all else. So naturally, going to this healing ministry created an inner conflict within.

Do I share my story and intentions with others? How, in the fervor and excitement of this trip, can I worry about what others think? Even in my strongest hour, I am still vulnerable to coveting other people's affirmation above yours, Lord. Please forgive me. I finally realized it really didn't matter what others thought. All that mattered is that I was following God's will, and I would move heaven and earth to help my son.

Joshy didn't understand why we were going on a trip, but he certainly was ecstatic to see the other airplanes and ride "Up, up, up in the sky!" We settled into our hotel and headed out that Saturday morning to attend the program at Dr. Wright's church. With a joyous heart, I truly believed complete and total healing was possible. I also believed that even if this ministry did not provide a pathway of spiritual healing for my son, I was going to remain humbled by the experience and thank the Lord for making me more aware of the spiritual healing that Scripture describes.

Luke 8:47 (KJV) describes the scene when the hemorrhaging woman touched the hem of Jesus garment:

> Now when the woman saw that she was not hidden, she came trembling; and falling down before Him, she declared to Him in the presence of all the people the reason she had touched Him and how she was healed immediately. And He said to her, "Daughter, be of good cheer; your faith has made you well. Go in peace."

HEALING BEGINS

The conference was hosted at Mount Pleasant Church in Macon, Georgia. It was a modest, but beautiful white church with a fellowship hall large enough to host a few hundred people. The initial group session, was quite lengthy, which was torturous for my restless little boy who only wanted to play. Finally, we were instructed to branch off into individualized meetings with two facilitators who were led by the Holy Spirit and trained in healing ministry. Initially we were paired with two women who were filled with compassion while they asked me candid questions about Joshy's struggles. I summarized Joshy's life story—his development, the ADHD, bipolar disorder, and auditory hallucinations.

While speaking in these generic terms, Joshy was calm and content as he casually played at our table. But the moment our conversation with the facilitators became more personal, Joshy's personality morphed before our very eyes. We witnessed a darkened aura sweep over his eyes as his entire body stiffened. His mood dramatically shifted, and he became agitated and depressed. Joshy's body literally recoiled into the corner of the wall and he started screaming, "Leave me alone! Leave me alone!"

His personality change thickened the air surrounding us, turning it stale. I looked toward the women with pleading eyes, praying they could help my son. They tried in earnest to get Joshy to be responsive to their questioning and prayers, but it wasn't working. Eventually the women stopped and suggested that perhaps Joshy would be more responsive to a male facilitator. While they were locating another facilitator, I urged Joshy to creep out from the corner of the room where he was cowering in a defensive position. As he slowly approached me, I reached my arms out and he latched on to my shoulders. His trembling body shook with fear as he buried his head into my chest; he tried to find solace which only my embrace could provide He was terrified, and it was my responsibility to comfort him. With a soothing voice I promised him that these people only wanted to help him be happy and know Jesus. Joshy stayed in the safety of my arms for the remainder of the session.

Joshy developed an instant rapport with the second attempt by the male facilitator. After a few minutes of play, the facilitator explained that he was there to help; he asked if he could offer up a simple prayer on Joshy's behalf. Joshy slowly nodded his head. He also asked Joshy if he would agree to repeat back the words of this special prayer. Joshy did not like this idea, but he finally relented with a huff, puff, and pouty lips.

Arms crossed, Joshy hesitantly began to repeat the man's prayer verbatim. I'm not sure he understood the enormity of what was happening, but I do believe that God changes hearts. At first Joshy had a reluctant, grumpy quality in his voice.

"Dear God." (Audible sigh.)

"It's me, Joshy." (Huge swallow.)

"I know you created me and love me." (Hhhmmmphh!)

His reluctance continued until we were about ten minutes into the prayer. At that point, finally all attitudes and distractions faded as Joshy became hyper-attuned. He suddenly closed his eyes and took ownership of the mighty words he prayed. It was astonishing to hear a strong, *clear*, passionate, emphatic voice burst out of my little boy. That day I was privileged to witness Joshy take ownership of his soul. He was smiling with peace and joy infiltrating his heart. Suddenly the most beautiful words I could have possibly heard emerged from Joshua's lips. His eyes were now wide and beaming while he rejoiced, "I *am* a child of God! Heal me Jesus! Make the voices go away, they are not yours. Fill me with your Holy Spirit! Amen!"

I started weeping as waves of what felt like delicate ladybugs washed over my skin. We were experiencing the Holy Spirit among us. The healing power of the Holy Spirit fell upon my precious child. We left the ministry ecstatic; we could not wait to see this supernatural change manifest itself within him back at home. He never did hear the voices again. They were obliterated, eradicated! He experienced complete and total healing of the voices.

During Joshy's first month home, the spiritual war raging within his soul had ceased. There was a peace in his eyes. No more tortured voices. Praise be to God! Because of this experience I now stand and proclaim that my son was once demon possessed and being tortured by voices, *but the Lord healed him*. Halleluiah! *This* experience was a testimony of God's faithfulness and healing power that He wanted me to share with others.

A MARRIAGE DIVIDED

We returned home walking on air. Victory! But it was short-lived because we quickly realized that although Joshy's voices were gone, there were still behaviors, tantrums, and developmental delays to contend with. After the high of the trip to Georgia wore off I slowly became discouraged again. I started to unjustly downplay the significance of Joshy's healing because I saw so many other obstacles ahead.

Lord, was I not specific enough down in Georgia? Doesn't praying for healing require You to provide a complete product? Is this only a partial healing? Is this some type of cruel joke? I don't think this is funny! Haven't we been through enough? Hasn't his little body and mind been stretched and pulled in enough ways already? How can you do this to us? How? It's not fair!

This negativity festered inside me, and it began to impact my relationship with Dave. We started fighting more frequently about our parenting skills, and the laughter in our home became minimal. I saw Dave treating Joshy differently than the other children. He was strict and determined to teach Joshy something with his tough love approach. This was hard for me to understand because his parenting approach was much more intense than the other aspects of his easy going personality with which I fell in love. I also didn't see that intensity when he was interacting with the other children, so I thought it wasn't fair. I was changing as well. While Dave was at work I found myself playing bad cop, screeching at the kids and doling out consequences. I would call Dave and plead with him to get home by five o'clock. Then he would leave his very important job and rush home to save me from the insanity, dreading what was to be in store when he walked through the door. By the time Dave came home, I switched off my mommy role, which left Dave with no choice but to fill my shoes. And then I had the audacity to judge his parenting methods. I morphed into a good cop; I became the mother bear protecting her cub. The disparity in our parenting styles was pervasive. I started picking my battles in my quest for peace and quiet. However, Dave continued to micromanage Joshy's every move and misbehavior, resulting in constant punishment such as time outs or loss of privileges.

⁂

One day we ventured into the hollows of our garage for some spring cleaning. Trying to teach our children to contribute to the family, Dave gave Joshy one little task. His job was to put the kite with its twenty five foot tail into a skinny plastic sheath. Dave told him what to do and then went somewhere else while I stood close by watching Joshy. Within ten minutes Joshy was in tears because he could not manipulate his hands to push the long tail into the plastic sheath.

Every fiber of my body was on high alert; I wanted to reach out and do this for him. I could have the job done in five seconds. Yet when Dave saw him crying, he sternly told Joshy that he *would* do this, and it didn't matter if it took all day. He *would* and he *could* do this. I was in tears; I thought Joshy needed a visual or hands-on demonstration to be successful, but Dave made it clear that I was not to help. I didn't want to defy my husband, but again, a mother bear's protection of her cubs supersedes all else. I agonized, watching Joshy struggle for thirty brutal, drawn-out minutes.

Finally I confronted Dave. I suggested that Joshy literally did not have the ability to do this because something was not processing between his brain, eyes, and hands. But Dave believed Joshy simply was not trying. Dave told him, "You just don't *want* to do it," but I wholeheartedly disagreed. I didn't see Joshy defying us and saying no, and he was not running away screaming. Instead he wept as he struggled to please his father.

Our divergent philosophies about Joshy's capabilities and limitations became glaringly obvious. *We used to be on the same page, Lord. What is happening to us?* I prayed. The more tasks Joshy struggled to accomplish, the harder Dave pushed him, and the more uncomfortable I became. Deep in Dave's heart, he loved Joshy immensely, he just really wanted him to succeed, and he hoped his son would have all the advantages life had to offer. But Dave and I were simply resorting to different styles of parenting due to the constant barrage of incidences like this.

I tried to cope by picking up literature on ADHD, bipolar disorder, and spiritual writings for inspiration. I became resentful toward Dave because I had an endless supply of information to share about Joshy's diagnoses, but he could not keep up with the literature I provided. I tried to plant the material near bathroom toilets and coffee tables. Nothing worked.

To my amazing husband's defense, I never told him the depths of my frustration over this because I was always avoiding confrontation. I figured he could read my mind and know how much I believed that reading these books was the number one priority for our family. Furthermore, Dave has always struggled with concentration when reading lengthy material. I could not understand how this seemingly minor difficulty could impede his desire to know every minute detail about what made his son tick. *I don't care if Dave commutes two hours a day and works sixty hours per week! He needs to get on my band wagon!* I fumed. My expectations were so ridiculous.

FIREWORKS

That summer we visited Dave's parents in Connecticut over the Fourth of July holiday. During the trip my resentments toward Dave reached their boiling point. I know I should have discussed my concerns with Dave earlier, but I was such a peacemaker (*or peacefaker*), I always avoided all possible confrontations. So I let my intense, negative feelings build up when instead I should have considered what Dave was going through. But this particular day I could not bear even one more second listening to Dave yell at Joshy, bestowing punishment upon punishment on him for his poor listening skills, noncompliance, or impulsive behaviors.

The explosion culminated that evening as we were walking down his parents' long driveway to the cul-de-sac below to watch the fireworks. Halfway down the driveway, Joshy had a mild indiscretion resulting in another punishment. This time Dave sent Joshy to wait in a bedroom back at the empty house all alone. Joshy was scared and bawling, and I was seething over the possibility that Joshy had to stay in an unoccupied house and that he might miss the fireworks. Although I wanted to correct Joshy's behavior as well, history had proven that disciplining Joshy *never* prevented the behavior from reoccurring. I felt Dave's consequence to be rash and out of proportion to the behavior.

I stormed off down the driveway with smoke pouring out my ears. As I confronted Dave, the rest of the family went to the bottom of the cul de sac. In the great, wide open, Dave and I had a colossal, knock-down, drag out, verbal war with each other. I was sobbing, to which Dave seemed unresponsive, thus making me cry even harder. *This is so humiliating! Dave's parents are waiting for us at the end of the driveway! They won't think we're perfect anymore!* I worried.

Our argument lasted about thirty minutes while my in-laws silently and patiently waited for us to duke it out. I ranted and raved about how mean he seemed with his constant punishments. I accused him of not truly understanding Joshy's disabilities. He angrily responded that he was never going to make a decision regarding Joshy again. It was all mine to figure out alone. It was an ugly and exhausting scene, but in the end we came to an agreement to try to meet each other half way. We also decided to pursue counseling back at home. Finally, we reminded each other of our commitment to our marriage and family. Hand in hand we made the embarrassing walk down the drive and met up with our family. They were very respectful, tentatively bestowing half-smiles upon us with questioning eyes. *Let the fireworks begin!*

Next, Dave and I sought spiritual counseling back in Pennsylvania with Pastor Tim, the associate pastor at our Evangelical Free Church. After working with Pastor Tim for a few months, we realized that to save ourselves and our marriage, we needed to heed the advice of Proverbs 4:23, "Above all else, guard your heart, for it is the wellspring of life." (NIV) I prayed for Dave to find the desire and ability to turn to the Bible more frequently for guidance and support, knowing this was the most powerful way he could guard his heart.

Pastor Tim also helped Dave and I create a consistent plan to help us present a united front when new situations arose. First, we agreed to not undermine the other in a moment of crisis. Instead, we would debrief the incident and discuss our thoughts immediately after.

We also agreed to talk privately about all of Joshy's misbehaviors before slamming the gavel onto the marble table distributing consequences. We passed our first challenge when Joshy, in a fit of anger, scribbled on the walls with crayons throughout the entire downstairs of our home. I held my cool and didn't even acknowledge the behavior until Dave came home. When Dave arrived, together we questioned Joshy about his feelings and motives, and made him participate late into the night cleaning the walls. Dave and I felt encouraged because we presented a united front and did not overreact with emotion.

Joshy's Fourth Birthday Letter

As you sleep during your nap (which you still take at the age of four), I am taking a moment to be awed by your development this past year. I reflect back and see God's handiwork in our lives. You have come so very far my little love!

Although you are only four, you have the body of a six-year-old. You definitely have your father's genes! You are gorgeous; you are absolutely stunning with your clear, hazel eyes, light hair, and dark tan.

Guess what? We thought you had ten cavities this year! You poor thing, we brushed and brushed your gums, only to find a new dentist who said your teeth looked excellent! You have such a great smile Joshy. You are getting much better at brushing your teeth. Although you usually prefer mommy to do things for you, I am trying to help you become more independent. You are starting to do lots of things on your own like washing your hands and face and taking a bath. Such accomplishments!

You still love food and Spiderman. You have also developed quite a singing voice this year. I am excited to see how this develops. My prayer is that one day you could use this for the Lord. Have I told you how wonderful you've been with your baby brother this year? Joshy, this year your heart has grown so much. You are the most endearing little boy; everyone thinks so! You were never jealous of Caleb; instead you welcomed him to our family with open arms. You are so protective of Caleb. Your heart amazes me.

You love intensely and feel emotions so intensely! You get so excited about things that we stopped telling you in advance about fun activities because otherwise the wait tortured you. You are so affectionate and loving. You have a way about you that can sense when somebody needs a hug.

You are wonderful.

I am very excited to see how God grows you in next year. Soon you will be in school, and Mommy's heart will be a little sad missing you every day. But I know He has great plans for you. I love you more than you'll ever know. You are my first born boy and I just love you to pieces. Love, Mommy

SEPARATION

That fall I opted to place Joshy in kindergarten as a young five-year-old. His summer birthday warranted us the option of either waiting an extra year or sending him to school early. I chose to send him early because frankly, he needed more therapy and stimulation, which I knew the school system could provide. One part of me believed that placing Joshy into kindergarten that year was an enormous mistake, yet my faith in God's will for our lives reminded me this decision was all part of His mighty plan. After all, Joshy's perilous experiences in kindergarten resulted in more answers and more help. But it had to get much worse for this to happen.

Joshy was placed in Mrs. Muffin's kindergarten classroom. I was nervous about this placement because she was an older teacher with one foot out the school door and into retirement. Before the year started I explained to Mrs. Muffin that Joshy might have difficulty and need some extra attention. Joshy was re-evaluated to determine if he would continue to qualify for special education services in the elementary school. Based upon observation and testing results, an updated IEP was crafted. Although the plan included weekly speech therapy and occupational therapy, there wasn't a formal behavioral plan.

Joshy's disruptive classroom behaviors included impulsivity that manifested by calling out of turn, poor voice modulation, and ignoring personal space. He also became easily frustrated and would cry daily when the work was too difficult. Oh how he wanted to fit in and make friends, to learn with the rest of his class! Unfortunately his emotional liability prevented adequate social and academic progress.

During the winter of kindergarten Joshy developed separation anxiety. At first I tried to ignore it and encourage him to go to school, yet he would only cling to me while screaming. I began to realize the desperation Joshy felt at the prospect of being separated from me. This behavior escalated one blustery winter day when the school bus picked him up the street at the corner.

Initially, Joshy started up the steps of the big bus and walked down the aisle at a glacial pace. When he glanced out the window and saw me waving goodbye, without warning he became hysterical. He climbed up over the seats, *on top of students* to fight his way back to the front door. I was stunned. He tore out of the bus door and started running down the road. I reached for him as he blew by me, and just barely snagged his winter jacket as he wildly ran away. He was frantically swinging his arms and legs, sending his shoes, jacket, and shirt flying into the air. My primary concern was for my son's safety and peace of mind, but I was also humiliated beyond belief having the entire neighborhood watch us like we were a spectacle in a three ring circus. Of course the bus had to leave.

In the meantime I chased my half-naked son down the icy, wintery road surface all the way back to our house. I was numb; I was on auto-pilot. I did *not* know what to do to help him! One thing I was darn sure of was that he was not going to win this battle. He *was going to school.* I mistakenly considered these incidents to be power struggles in which I was determined to win. I lost touch with the depth and gravity of Joshy's mental illness. Joshy was truly terrified of the world. There was never a winner in the end.

The separation anxiety continued on a daily basis. One morning when I hauled Joshy into school after he missed the bus, I confided in Mrs. Muffin about how difficult it was to coax him onto the bus. In that moment, with downcast eyes void of any hope for the future, she said, "It's is such a shame." *You are an awful, witchy woman, I don't want your pity!* I thought. I would have pulled Joshy from the class if there was another option. Her cruel ignorance toward my son's mental illness ignited an awareness that the Easton area school district was officially lacking in sensitivity training for their teachers. I started driving Joshy to school every morning, as I just couldn't let another serious bus incident occur. Luckily they had a drive-up line where the teacher or principal would escort them into the school doors nearby. This new method worked for a few weeks, but quickly his anxiety and trepidation returned with a vengeance.

CRESCENDO

Joshua's anxiety culminated one morning when I pulled up to the drop off line at school. He started whimpering and screaming as he refused to step out of the car. I calmly told him this was unacceptable behavior and that he *must* get out of the car. No response and icy eyes locked upon mine ready for a showdown. Dreading what was likely to transpire, I walked to the other side of the car to personally escort him out, yet he resisted with all his might.

As I turned my head to see the staff just standing there staring at us, Joshy suddenly leapt out of the car and dashed across the busy parking lot. With so many half-asleep, unsuspecting drivers, I feared for his life. Instinctively I scrambled after him and proceed to jump on top of him, planting him face down on the pavement. All the mothers, bus drivers, teachers, and the principal stared at us in shock and judgment. I covered Joshy with my body and prayed for the Lord to calm him. After a few minutes I could not block the car line any longer. I promised him that I would enter the school building with him and would not leave.

Holding hands, we managed to get as far as the principals' office. Once inside, I started to negotiate my departure again. But the mere mention of me leaving sent Joshy into another tailspin. Joshy started throwing items in the office and was cowering in fear under the principal's chair. Next, he ran into the hallway and began wailing at the top of his lungs.

The principal became frantic and agitated as well, so he started screaming at me, "I can't have him disrupt my entire school! If you don't control your son now, *I'm calling the police!*" It stopped me in my tracks. I could not fathom his ludicrous threat to call the police on a five-year-old child. Joshy was clearly out of his mind. He was sick, and he was terrified; he didn't know what he was doing. I was frantic and embarrassed; I started to fall apart in front of the school administrators who gathered to watch helplessly in the foyer. Finally, the nurse gently led me into her office and suggested that I consider crisis intervention services. Handing me a phone book, she explained that there were inpatient treatment centers scattered throughout Pennsylvania. This nurse angel allowed me to sit at her desk and make calls to try and find a facility that would help my little one.

I quickly learned there was minimal availability for what they called a bed at a pediatric facility. Most programs would not take a five-year-old, and those that did had a waiting list a mile long. But I knew Joshy desperately needed help so I persevered. Two hours and twenty calls later, with most of my time spent on hold, I finally hit the jackpot with Friends Children's Hospital based in Philadelphia. I knew nothing about the facility or their credentials; I was grasping at straws on automatic pilot and blind faith. Meanwhile, Dave rushed out of work and headed home so that we could drive Joshy down for an emergency assessment together.

FRIENDS

Friends Hospital was far away and for first timers like us, it was intimidating. It felt like we were driving to a funeral. On the ride down, I asked Joshy if he knew why he was going to a hospital and whether he remembered what happened at school earlier. Amazingly, he did not remember a single thing. I described the harrowing details in an attempt to jog his memory but nothing worked. The incidence was so extreme and traumatic that Joshy blocked it from his consciousness. When I glanced back into those hazel-yellow eyes, he looked exhausted.

At the hospital we sat in a tiny room for three hours and waited for impressions from the assessment team. Eventually they returned and recommended inpatient hospitalization. Dave and I somberly stared at each other in disbelief. My heart was constricting as I realized the scope of Joshy's sickness; I was sending my five year-old-son away from every comfort and the love of his family to help him get well. Joshy's original fears of separation and abandonment were coming true. I feared he would think we were rejecting him and that he could not understand the depth of our love. I was consumed with anger at God, guilt for my weaknesses, and grief over his lost childhood.

When we finally admitted Joshy, it was eleven at night, and we were exhausted. The psychiatric program was in an old, decrepit wing of hospital; I was reluctant to leave him. The living conditions were utterly horrendous. The scratched and dented walls were painted a sick orange, and the carpets reeked of urine. I shuddered at the thought of him getting ready in his stenchy, cold bathroom. I complained to staff about the conditions, but they placated me, explaining that these hospital conditions were actually better than others! Wow. I prayed the quality of care was far superior to the substandard environment.

Joshy's bedroom included four empty walls, an unmade bed, and one dresser. There was nothing to soothe or comfort him! I prayed like his life depended on it:

> Lord, Please do not give him a roommate. He's the youngest child here! I fear an older, aggressive child could hurt him. Please let the quality of care be far superior to this dirty environment. Take away his fears, Lord. Please don't let him cry when we leave. How long will he have to be here? Why is this happening to him, why?

Despite my best attempts to describe the pain I endured, it is impossible. The banality of the English language falls short with its limited descriptors. Only Scripture comes close to adequately portraying this turmoil in Psalm 55:21: (NIV)

> My heart is in anguish within me; the terrors of death assail me; Fear and trembling have beset me; horror has overwhelmed me. I said "Oh that I had the wings of a dove! I would flee far away and stay in the desert; I would hurry to my place of shelter far from the tempest and the storm.

I could relate to that verse. When my heart was in anguish I felt like the little girl Jenny in the movie Forrest Gump (1994) who wanted to be like a bird so she could fly "far, far away." I would do anything to escape the pain; soaring above the adversity below sounded perfect.

Although I was an emotional wreck throughout Joshy's ten day treatment in Philly, I had to admit that I enjoyed the peaceful house as life became simpler. Alexa and Caleb were flourishing from some much deserved attention, and after the first two nights I caught up on my sleep. But I still couldn't make the vivid images of the deplorable conditions my baby was surrounded by go away.

We were required to visit the hospital every few days for a team meeting. Upon arrival my heart would leap out of my chest when I would catch that first glimpse of my little guy racing down the hallway ready to jump into my arms. We would nuzzle into each other's necks and I swear I never wanted to let go. But the inevitable goodbye that soon followed was full of grief and despair. *Dear Lord, does Joshy think we don't love him and are sending him away for being a bad boy?* I prayed.

GLORY TO GOD

It was difficult not to become self absorbed in what I was going through. I started to feel and behave like a martyr; my sole identity became "Jamie Bierut, mother of a special needs child and struggling every day." I played the woe-is-me act to perfection. I bought an unnecessarily large house, overindulged when shopping, and compulsively indulged in food because I thought I deserved it due to my struggles. Little did I realize that my indulgences were only bringing more hardship upon myself after that short term high of getting what I hoped would make me feel better. I wanted everybody to know Joshy's sad story, and I wanted to be rewarded and noticed for my pain.

But praise God, His Holy Spirit is stronger than my narcissism! I finally sought refuge in verses Psalm 71: 20-21: (NIV) "Though you have made me see troubles, many and bitter, you *will* restore my life again; from the depths of the earth you *will* increase my honor and comfort me once again." This promise enabled me to greet each morning and muddle through the day. I was also strengthened by my sweet Christi, far away in Indiana:

> Dearest Jamie, I just got up. God was doing a "thing" with me again last night, and I didn't get to sleep until five thirty. I was up from about midnight to two thirty reading the Word and writing down what came to my heart. When I awoke this morning, there were words in my head again. This time, it was this: I didn't actually hear any audible voice to recognize who it was. It was more these words specifically, but someone was praying for Joshy to be healed. I heard the prayer, but not the voice: the impression on my soul of exact words. The

words that answered the prayer were specifically this: *"I am using Joshy to bring glory to My Name."* What impressed me most was the emphasis on the present time. This message is in the here and now. God's very present purpose is being played out today, though it may be hard to see and even harder to feel in the difficulty of the moment and the fatigue of the day, and the questioning, questioning, questioning…Joshy is in the Lord's hand. And he IS bringing Gory to the Name of the *Most High God.* Isn't that a beautiful blessing upon your child?

In Mark 10 Jesus reminds us the value of his children. "Let the children come to me for the Kingdom of God belongs to such as they. Don't send them away!" Joshy belongs to Jesus. When he says, "Don't send them away," there are two ways to send (or cast) someone away: from your physical presence, and/or from your heart. It is important to pray that the Lord will keep Joshy close to your heart, and remain precious to your heart always. Know that you are in God's hand and in His heart today.

Love, Christi.

I was also lifted up in prayer by my mighty prayer warriors covering the states of Indiana, Ohio, Connecticut, Pennsylvania, and Virginia. Utilizing new technology and the internet enabled the power of prayer through strangers! It was a humbling and overwhelming blessing. Over time I have learned to embrace the spiritual gifts God has bestowed upon me, but deep inside I coveted the blessed gift of intercessory prayer given to others. Since it was not my strength, I was most grateful to these soldiers of prayer.

A NEW DIRECTION

Toward the end of Joshy's stay at Friends, the treatment team called a meeting to discuss Joshy's progress. During this meeting I was introduced to the term pervasive developmental disorder-NOS (PDD-NOS). I knew what this diagnosis meant, but I could not believe they attached this to my own child. The DSM-IV recognizes this diagnosis only when there is a severe and pervasive impairment in the development in reciprocal social interaction or verbal and nonverbal communication skills, or when stereotyped behavior, interest, and activities are present but the child does not meet full criteria for any other developmental disorder, such as autism (American Psychiatric Association, 2000). *I can't believe these doctors really think my child is on the high end of the autistic spectrum?*I thought.

Exasperated, the disbelief flooded my veins; I could not handle another diagnosis! My first question to the psychiatrist was, "Does this mean Joshy doesn't have the other diagnoses anymore?"

"Actually, we think he still meets the diagnostic criteria for ADHD, but the prior bipolar diagnosis is really just behaviors manifested within PDD-NOS. "

"Why wasn't this discovered until now? I have been trying to find answers for years!"

"Sometimes it takes a few years for each child's developmental delays to become more substantial. The past few years, Joshua's delays have become more apparent. You should consider yourselves lucky that we have discovered this at an early age. This allows us to intervene accordingly right away."

I didn't feel lucky; I felt confused and skeptical. Regardless of this latest diagnosis, the one thing I knew for certain was that *nothing was different.* Joshy remained the love of my life. He was the same delightful little boy who could still bring me joy amidst the hardship.

When we arrived a few days later for Joshy's release, he flew into our arms as we showered him with hugs and kisses. We promised him this was a new beginning and that we would do everything possible to make sure he never had to go away again. The hospital's recommendations at discharge were for a neurological consultation at Children's Hospital in Philadelphia (CHOP), outpatient psychiatry sessions, and Provider 50 Wrap Around Services. Provider 50 was a comprehensive, state-funded program that offered intensive services comprised of a home-based behavior specialist, a mobile therapist, and a therapeutic support specialist. Friends also changed Joshy's medications; he entered the unit taking Risperdal, Depakote, and Concerta, but he was leaving with Concerta and a new, unfamiliar drug called Moban.

The only information I was given at the hospital in regard to the Moban was that he *must* receive his dose at consistent intervals throughout the day. Furthermore, they did not give us any pills to take home, and there was no pharmacy available at the hospital to fill the prescription on a Friday night. We raced home anyway, nothing could dampen our elation. We returned to home sweet home where we had decorated the kitchen with streamers, bought his favorites toys, and had cake and ice cream waiting to celebrate his return.

MOBAN

The next morning was Saturday, and two things were on the agenda. First, we wanted to reacclimate Joshy to our home routine, and second, we had to fill the Moban prescription. Dave drove to the local pharmacy around nine in the morning, but he returned empty handed.

"Dave, what happened? Why don't you have it?"

"The pharmacy said they don't carry this medication, and they would have to order it. It can't get here until Monday."

"Monday? Are you serious?"

Dave suggested we call other local pharmacies to see if it was available elsewhere. My anxiety started rising as the clock's tick-tick became louder by the second, reminding me the little time we had until his next dose. At this point we were uneducated about Moban; all we knew was the doctors said Joshua *must* take this dose as scheduled. *Is he going to crash without it? Is he going to spontaneously combust or something?* An hour later, after calling all pharmacies within the Easton/Bethlehem area, we were out of luck. None of them could get the drug until Monday as well, which just wasn't soon enough. In the meantime he was due for his dose at eleven.

Two more hours passed, and now my anxiety turned into a full blown panic. Heart racing and tears flowing, we widened our geographical search for potential pharmacies. *Does anybody in this country carry this medication?* I agonized. I should have known right then that there was something foreboding about this drug. Finally, we found a pharmacy *an hour away* in Allentown. With adrenaline flowing, I set off in the car on a mission to get the Moban. Joshua's next dose was over an hour late, but mercifully he was fine. After this mishap, we established the prescription at our local pharmacy as a monthly necessity to prevent this from ever happening again. What we didn't know was that Joshy would only be taking Moban for a few weeks.

I sat down one night and started to research this this mysterious drug. I learned that Moban was approved for the treatment of schizophrenia nearly thirty-eight years ago. I also learned that Moban works by blocking the effects of the neurotransmitter dopamine, which in turn decreases delusions and hallucinations. Moban could also reduce hyperactivity and aggressiveness (Molindone, 2011). Over the years doctors started prescribing it for mood disorders as well with moderate success.

But Moban also caused some extremely dangerous side effects. Studies have indicated that there were increased mortality rates in elderly patients being treated with Moban. Furthermore, there was potential for a severe side effect called tardiv dyskinesia, and Joshy fell victim to this tragic condition. Tardiv dyskinesia presents as repetitive, involuntary, and purposeless movements that include grimacing, tongue protrusion, lip smacking, puckering and pursing of the lips, and rapid eye blinking (http://www.tardive-dyskinesia.com/index.html, June 20, 2011).

JERKS & TWITCHES

The first thing I noticed was that Joshy was doing something weird with his tongue. He looked like a frog trying to catch flies in his mouth; his tongue would spontaneously burst forth from his lips as if he was catching a lollipop floating by in the air. His attempts to keep his tongue inside his mouth were entirely out of his control. He also started flexing his fingers spontaneously in different directions. They never stopped moving.

Then the most debilitating symptom emerged: he started having spasms in his neck and limbs, accompanied by erratic emotions and agitation. The spasms became progressively worse over a three day period until one day Joshy could not stand, sit, or speak. It was horrifying to watch! He vacillated between jerking wildly, falling down, and flopping out of chairs. If he tried to stand, his legs would kick out and buckle. His head would crick to the right, his arms would literally fly up into the air for no reason. It was clear Joshy was in a medical crisis. We raced back to the Lehigh Valley Emergency Room.

This trip to the ER was gut wrenching. The medical staff just stood by and watched Joshy suffer; there was little they could do to alleviate his agony. The Cogentin they administered to counteract the involuntary muscle spasms proved ineffective. The doctors tried a shot of Benadryl, but again, this had no effect.

As midnight approached I realized Joshy had been convulsing for sixteen hours. *Lord, please give Joshy some rest, I beg of you!* I was dying inside. I pleaded with the Lord to give me Joshy's pain, but He didn't grant me this wish. I really would have embraced all his pain and suffering if Joshua could be spared. After three hours of observation, they doctors informed me there was nothing they could do. They refused to touch Joshy with a ten foot pole because of his complicated mental health history. Worse yet, they kept stressing the potential permanency of tardiv dyskinesia (like I needed any reminding!) The staff offered a consolation prize of one Ativan pill to help his body to calm down enough to sleep. But one Ativan did not do the trick, so I had to give him a second dose on the car ride home.

Late that night as I drove down the highway, his weary body finally gave in to the Ativan and blessed sleep fell upon him. Exhausted, I cried out in anguish to God. I didn't understand how He could allow Joshy to continue to be plagued in so many ways! Was it a punishment for my own sins being manifested in Joshy? I didn't have *any* answers, and it drove me insane. I cursed Moban's very existence and Friend's Hospital for prescribing such an archaic drug.

On the drive home while I ranted and raved to God, Carrie Underwood's song "Wasted" (2005) was playing on the radio. Crying my eyes out, I focused on the following verse:

> I don't wanna spend my life jaded, waiting to wake up
> one day and find, that I've let all these years go by wasted.
> I ain't spending no more time wasted.

I was screaming the lyrics, my own agony spewing forth in these words. I looked in the backseat and saw my resting child, and made a commitment right then to take him off all medications. They simply were making him worse. I didn't want to drug my child to the point of sedating him throughout his childhood. I only wanted to help improve the quality of his life.

MOMMY TAKES THE DRIVER'S SEAT

My career always spiraled between work and home. It seemed as soon as I settled into the working world, circumstances with Joshy would change and I would need to resign. Full time employment during his early years was simply out of the question. Yet as he reached school age I yearned for the socialization and stimulation a part time job could provide. I even tried my own business and I worked for Crayola's "Big Yellow Box" business as an independent consultant. Although I was very successful consultant it started taking away from too much family time. After Joshy's hospitalization it was clear that my business meant nothing compared to my son's well being. I resigned and focused all my energy on Joshy's health.

The first step was to take Joshy off all his medication over the next few weeks. It was time to become his sole advocate and make decisions based on a mother's gut instinct and guidance from God. Despite years of insecurities as a mother, I finally realized that God had equipped me with compassion, intelligence, and resourcefulness to prepare me for this very day. With confidence I suggested and administered medications, coordinated doctors' appointments and psychiatry appointments, followed up on speech and occupational therapy, and navigated the school system. For example, now that Moban was no longer needed at school, I comprised a letter to update his teacher and nurse on his medical status:

Wedneday, April 26, 2006

To: Mrs. Mainzer, "Nurse Dee," Mrs. Goldsmith

I needed to update you on Joshua's current medical and psychiatric situation. Last week we learned some disturbing news that a medication Joshua was taking after his stay at Friend's Hospital could lead to a serious neurological condition known as tardiv dyskinesia. Consequently, we immediately started weaning him from the medicine. To make a very long story short, the symptoms have continued despite stopping the medication. This manifests as tics, purposeless movement, and tremors. This is also paired with major agitation and frustration, of course. This condition could be permanent.

Although the condition is often reversible, since Tuesday, we have already seen incredible improvement. However, he is still unable to perform some basic activities of daily living (eating, brushing teeth). I am not sure how he will function in the school environment, but he desperately wants to come back to school despite the fact that he does not have the motor coordination to even write his name. The spasms have decreased to the point that other children will not notice. Therefore, I have made the decision to bring him back to class today with the understanding that if there are any problems, you will not hesitate to call me immediately so I can come and pick him up. If he continues to greatly struggle at school we can discuss our options later.

Therefore, as of Thursday, April 25, Joshy will not be taking Moban or Concerta as listed in his medical file. We are ceasing all medication at this time and hope with vigilant Provider 50 services we may not need to restart them in the future. I realize that discontinuing the Concerta may cause Joshy to have greater difficulty with sustained concentration and activity level. Please notify me if this becomes unmanageable. Thank you for the care and compassion you extend upon my child. God bless.

I was on pins and needles waiting to see how Joshy would handle his transition back to kindergarten. Luckily the school nurse was very supportive and helped me arrange an incentive for him upon arrival. I agreed to drive Joshy to school, enter a quiet side door, and escort him directly to the nurse's office. There he could find a giant bag of candy waiting for his chubby fingers to filter through. If he transitioned into the building without incident, he would pick a candy of choice. Since Joshy's reason for living centered around sweet treats the candy was the perfect motivator. Our plan was immediately successful enabling me to leave him at school without having anxiety about his adjustment.

The classroom was a different story. His teacher was not equipped to handle an under medicated, inattentive, hyperactive, socially delayed child. She did not provide him with the assistance he required to engage appropriately with the other students. Although he did complete those last few months of kindergarten without incident, there was minimal to no academic or social progress. But I knew it was worth it in order to give him a break from the medication.

To Medicate or Not To Medicate

As much as I despised Friend's Hospital for what ensued with Joshy, at least this travesty was the catalyst that started intensive, home-based, therapeutic services. The good news was that I was finally going to get some help at home with my son. But the bad news was that we were mandated to find another psychiatrist and another blasted psychological assessment to pursue these services.

After such treacherous results from prior medication trials, we were reluctant to try any other medications. I spent days and nights praying and thinking about my stance on psychiatric medicine and whether it was in Joshua's best interests. When deciding to medicate, the risk of side effects is extensive and varied. But when the risk of not doing something is greater than the risks of the medication itself, I ultimately opted to medicate. Suicide or self injurious behaviors are a far greater risk than the side effects of most drugs. Many parents are scared to medicate their children. Some think that agreeing to medicate is a reflection of their inability to parent their child. Others think they are poisoning or sedating their child. I know this type of thinking, for I have twisted my motives and wondered these things for years.

Through much prayer and counsel, I have learned to try natural alternatives first, and if that proves unsuccessful, then consider other means. Properly medicating a child who is suffering utilizes a resource which God has gifted us. Please do not feel guilty when helping your child requires medication! If your child had diabetes would you give them insulin to survive?

It is the same with mood disorders. If a chemical is missing from the brain which results in suffering, don't we need to respond with appropriate medication as well? It was not easy to know when Joshua's needs were bigger than what family supports, supplements, therapy, and the school system could provide. Every time I was faced with that decision I had to be brutally honest with myself and ask two critical questions.

First, was Joshy a danger to himself or others? Joshua was rarely a danger to others. Sometimes he would flail on the floor, wildly swinging his arms and legs. Other times he would kick or throw things. It would have been easier to ignore the behavior and pray the tantrums didn't last long, but I had to address God's standard of acceptable behavior in our home. I could ignore him and take the easy way out, but in my heart I knew the easy way out would only manifest in a massive problem down the road. But typically he just internalized all of the frustration and pain and struggled to utilize appropriate coping mechanisms. Trying to find his own way to punish himself, he would punch his thighs and bang his head into furniture.

Joshy's tendency to internalize negative feelings provided opportunities for me to remind him that although we all make mistakes, we can forgive each other like Christ forgives us. I showed him Psalm 103:12 (NLT) "He has removed our sins as far as the east is from the west."

Second, was Joshy suffering? Just thinking of the second question tugged at my emotions. At first it was difficult to decipher the difference between an ordinarily difficult day and when his pain ran deeper into the crevice of his heart and soul. But I slowly learned that beyond my own pain and survival, I had to stop and take a deep breath in order for me to truly see what was standing before me. Often I found a little boy who was scared, exhausted, and vulnerable. I found a confused, emotional child who did not understand what was happening to him. I saw great suffering.

Looking beyond his defiance and intensity, I could see a longing to escape the pain. He longed to have friends and play cooperatively with siblings. I saw a little boy who needed an incredible amount of help to feel safe in his unpredictable world. I had to take away all of my hurt and fatigue and focus only on his moments. I also had to be realistic about my own capabilities and resources. I had to acknowledge that I had other precious children to raise.

Since my answers to the two original questions were, "Yes he can be a danger to himself or others," and "Yes he is suffering," I cautiously proceeded with another psychiatrist. That spring I made oodles of phone calls covering the eastern quadrant of Pennsylvania hoping to find a good match. Finally, I stumbled upon what I considered to be the best of the best in private psychiatry—Dr. Zimmerman.

Dr. Zimmerman was the first doctor to ever sit down with us and eliminate our confusion. He drew out a tree grid on paper which helped to organize and simplify our areas of concern.

Together we created several branches on this tree which identified our top priorities (mood regulation, ADHD symptoms, social skills, etc.). He helped us accept that we could only address one area at time in order to be 100 percent certain of the impact of a new medication. We chose mood stabilization first. In the meantime, I scheduled this mandatory psychological assessment with Dr. Kaplan. Back in Easton our family of five clustered into a small, humid, empty room. After two hours of questioning, I mentally checked out; I was getting really sick of repeating every minute detail of our lives for the fiftieth time.

Dr. Kaplan agreed that Joshy and the entire family could benefit from Provider 50 services offered through Kids' Interventions Developmental Support Services (KIDSS). The intervention plan the agency crafted was a treasured gift that I clung to until our departure from Pennsylvania. They developed a plan that provided solutions for anger control, mood regulation, problem solving skills, transitioning, compliance, sibling conflict, social skills, and communication. Most of all, they strived to empower me to help Joshy in these areas. The icing on the cake—it was all free! *Thank you Jesus!*

With a referral in hand for a pediatric neurological consultation in Philadelphia, I was dismayed to learn it was going to take nearly nine months for an initial appointment. *Dear Lord, please help my child now!* I prayed. I fretted until I finally took action into my own hands. I begged, pleaded, and even tried to bribe the clerical staff with homemade brownies if they could sneak in an appointment for Joshy. Sure enough, one kind lady took pity upon me and slipped Joshy in a mere two days later! I detested being that squeaky wheel. It took so much of my energy, but there was no other way to get my son what he deserved.

The neurology team thoroughly examined Joshua and ordered many futile tests in an effort to rule out possible diagnoses that could have explained his developmental delays. The genetic testing proved negative for fragile x syndrome, the chromosomal array was unremarkable, MRI brain scans indicated normal impressions, and the EEG ruled out seizures. It seemed like we were on a never ending quest, circling endlessly round and round, never meant to find the answers. I wondered when I would ever be able to stop searching for answers, and if I could ever feel peace without knowing what was causing Joshua's problems.

BEHAVIOR MANAGEMENT

Once we agreed to pursue Provider 50 Services (a no-brainer), the agency swept into our home. A behaviorist was at my house nearly every day of the week, including Saturdays. Initially the lead clinician came out, and together we created Joshy's treatment plan. This was a comprehensive, sixteen page document that included a crisis plan, intervention methods, and benchmarks attached to goals. Their ideas were refreshing, and it helped me focus on being a proactive parent rather than a hopeless parent.

One of the first things we established was a snack system and schedule because Joshy begged for sweets every fifteen minutes. Typically I said no to these demands and then dealt with the aftermath. The snack schedule effectively reduced the tantrums, resulting in less conflict. I spent about a hundred dollars in supplies the first week. Purchases included tons of Velcro, poster boards, a three-tiered snack chest, markers, picture icons, construction paper, and glue.

The plastic snack chest was divided by drawers into healthy snacks and junk food snacks. I printed large icons that I attached outside each drawer. Next, I loaded the drawers with many nutritional options. I taught Joshy that snacks needed to be regulated and nutritious; he could have a snack every two hours between meals, but they must alternate between a healthy snack and a junk food choice. This worked marvelously and gave Joshy a small sense of control in his great big world. It stopped his constant yammering for snacks. Instead he wanted to know the time every fifteen minutes, but this was still improvement!

The second thing we established was that Joshy needed significant structure to his day, which could be achieved through a simple time and activities chart. His world was a scary, unpredictable world, so this schedule enabled him to see his entire day at a glance to alleviate surprises. The staff helped me create his personal schedule inside a manila folder. On the left there were three strips of Velcro running vertically, and on the right there were multiple strips running horizontally. The clinician laminated pictures and symbols to represent different activities scheduled throughout his day.

Joshy's responsibility was to choose from the reservoir of icons every night before bedtime in anticipation of the following day. These activities were placed in the left vertical column. First I would post some basic activities or errands, and then we would schedule in free play, room time, or chores. Once that was created, Joshy had the opportunity to pick from the reservoir of icons on the other page to choose exactly what he wanted to do during free play or room time. He placed these icons on the right vertical column. He had over a hundred options, including things like trampoline, walk in the park, and TV time.

I also came up with a three-foot-tall behavior board. I was really proud of this because I incorporated our faith and family values into it. There were five questions on the board that we reviewed twice a day. Using a similar Velcro system, Joshy would place a smiley, neutral, or sad face each morning and evening as we reflected upon his behavior. It was very important that Joshy took ownership and chose the face.

For each question I had a Bible quote underneath it. I wanted the children to know that our family's morals were not simply just because but to understand that this was the Lord's instruction for our lives. For example, one question listed was, "Did I have gentle hands today?" Then underneath it I quoted in big colorful letters Paul's first letter to Thessalonica, 2:7,

"We were gentle among you, like a mother caring for her little children."

Executing these new behavior strategies and witnessing Joshy's improvement was inspiring and empowering. The only glitch was the implementation of these strategies took *all* my time. And as grateful as I was for the interventionists who came over each day, I started feeling smothered. I had no time to myself in a house that I could no longer call my own. I knew I initially needed direction from KIDSS, but I did not want my hand held a moment longer than necessary. God blessed my family by providing these angels to equip and empower me.

After a few months, KIDSS involvement became more peripheral as I was gaining confidence. I networked resources with other mothers and any stranger I met along the way. I learned more about the autism spectrum and sought alternative treatments to help with some of the symptoms. I tried eliminating food dyes. I tried eliminating gluten. I tried removing extra yeast from his system by placing him on the probitiotics like acidophilus. I even took Joshy to music therapy.

LITHIUM

Things were looking brighter. The psychiatrist had a conservative plan that we embraced. Dave and I agreed to try another class of medications (antidepressants) before we resorted to standard treatment for mood stabilization—Lithium. First Joshy started a low dose of the antidepressant Lexapro. His response was similar to when he took stimulants. The desired effect was immediate; he was calmer, quieter, and more focused. However, within a few days his mood became erratic, swinging between frenzied, agitated, and desperate all before he ate his breakfast!

I came to learn these frequent mood vacillations were called ultradian cycling. Rapid cycling is when "children have frequent spikes and lows within a twenty-four-hour period." When this happens, their temperament and behavior become inflexible, oppositional, irritable, and explosive (Dimitri Papolos M.D. & Janice Papolos, 2006). I could only imagine how horrific and exhausting it must feel to alternate between extreme highs and lows *fifty* times a day.

Due to Joshy's rapid cycling, we discontinued the Lexapro after two weeks and prayed about our decision to try Lithium. I was anxious about the prospect of placing him on this drug. Despite its effectiveness at mood stabilization, it was notorious for its side effects to the thyroid and kidneys.

I asked Dr. Zimmerman, "What will happen to him if we give him this medicine but he's truly not bipolar?"

"If his body needs the Lithium, he will feel better. If you or I took Lithium and our bodies did not need it, we would feel sick and lethargic. If that happens for Joshua, we will stop immediately because his body doesn't need it."

I cannot describe the hours of sleep lost those nights, agonizing over the right choice. Ultimately I turned to Isaiah 30:21 "Whether you turn to the right or to the left, your ears will hear a voice behind you, saying, 'This is the way; walk in it.'" Finally clarity enveloped me and helped me see that there was no right or wrong turn on this journey; God would have my back in either direction.

Eventually Dave and I placed one step in front of the next and trusted this psychiatrist and our heavenly Father with blind faith. Getting Joshy's Lithium level to a therapeutic range took about one month. Typically people do experience mood stabilization the first month. But for Joshy, we saw results in two weeks! All of a sudden, he lost his edge. The little things that bothered him rolled off his back seamlessly. He didn't have that brittle reactivity (an overreaction to minor circumstances) anymore. My son was actually laughing and engaging with his brother and sister in an appropriate way. His cycles were stretching out. His mood changes were no longer occurring every half hour; instead, he was able to settle into a specific temperament which lasted all morning.

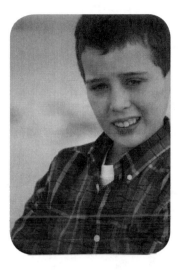

Joshua, eleven-years-old, winter 2012

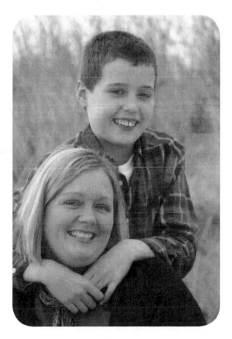

Joshua, eleven-years-old, with Mom at
Plymouth Beach on a warm winters day, winter 2012

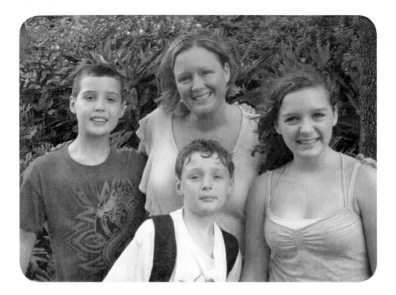

Joshua (11), Caleb "Boo" (8), Alexa (13),
and Mom at Sea World for spring break 2012

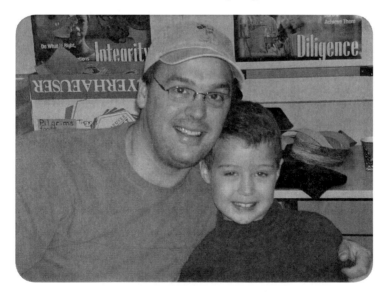

Dad and Joshua, eight-years-old, bonding at father-son night at
Plymouth's West Elementary CARE Program, winter 2009

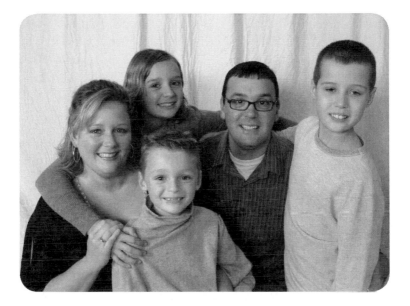

Family portrait, winter 2010, Mom, Alexa (11),
Caleb (6), Dad, Joshua (9)

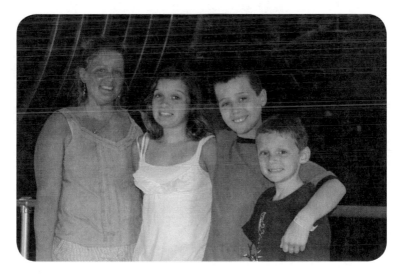

Mom, Alexa (12), Joshua (10), and Caleb (7),
spring break 2011 at the Houston Space Center

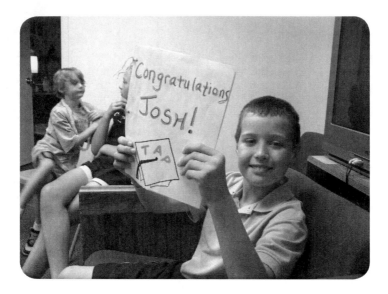

Joshua (9), summer 2010, graduation day from the TAP program

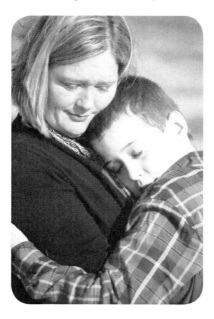

Joshua (11), safe in his mother's arms,
a refuge through the storms of life

PART 3

EAST COAST OASIS

Joshy was really growing up! At the age of five, I saw my little baby changing before my eyes as my chubby cheeked preschooler turned into a handsome young student ready to embrace the world. Naturally, about this time, we started calling him by his full name, Joshua. When he was five-years-old and the country was at the height of its economy, the inevitable financial crash was looming. Large companies such as Dave's employer Johnson & Johnson were among the first businesses to announce that significant layoffs were a certainty. With Dave's current position in jeopardy, he immediately started looking for work.

Dave had earned his outstanding reputation in the corporate world as a personable, creative, kind, and highly effective businessman. So it came as no surprise when he received two offers in one week. We were blessed to have one offer from Crayola in Easton, and the other from Genzyme in Cambridge, Massachusetts. While it would have been so much easier to stay in Easton, our priority was to seek God's will for our lives and provide stability for our family. Readily we opened our hearts to the idea of Massachusetts. Finally God was leading us toward an oasis.

Although I never minded moving, it was heartbreaking to leave my family and friends. I understood that Dave was our primary provider, and that I needed to support his journey. It was easier to embrace the new adventure knowing that I was never alone and that I could find happiness anywhere because God was always at my side. Happiness took a hiatus during our time in Pennsylvania, but I was determined to bring it back to life in Plymouth, Massachusetts.

We toured Boston and the south shore a few times, and I immediately fell in love with the ocean. We chose to settle in Plymouth. Although east coast living was considerably more expensive than the Midwest (we had several heart attacks when house hunting due to the inflation), we found that Plymouth had the most reasonably priced housing and offered a direct commuter rail into Boston. We were certain Plymouth was our new home based on the public schools' fantastic reviews, activities for families and children, and the beautiful landscape.

We chose a small, contemporary home. I fell in love with its cape-style architecture set against the backdrop of beautiful pines and a shimmering pond. I was in awe that my home was in one of the most historical towns in the country, on the edge of a natural forest, yet only five minutes away from the beach and waterfront. I felt like I had been waiting for Plymouth my entire life without knowing it. Good things were in store for us here; I could feel it from head to toe!

New Beginnings

We moved to Plymouth during August 2006 before the school year began, but the sale of our new home was not scheduled for closing until a month later. Consequently, our family of five needed to live in a hotel for four weeks until the closing date. We were blessed that Dave's company paid for our temporary accommodations at a local hotel. We tried to consider it a vacation, but it was really difficult due to such limited space. We crammed into one bedroom at night with the kids lying on air mattresses, piled into the tiny space like sardines in a can. Every morning we woke up itching from flea bites. Apparently the little critters were feasting each night while we slept in the dirty hotel room. It was disgusting!

Yet I was amazed at how well Joshua did with this transition. As long as his family was beside him every step of the way, he was able to go with the flow. It seemed that life changing events were easier for Joshua to handle than the minor daily variants.

Within a few days of hotel living, I resolved that I would *never* stay in this dark, moldy room unless I was sleeping. After school each day I picked up the kids from school and headed for a new beach. The beach was new and exciting every night. Perhaps the most amazing, magical, beach trip occurred when we visited White Horse Beach.

We frolicked in the warm sea and played on the clean strips of white sand. The tide was very low, and suddenly we started to see tiny holes spurting water from below the sand's surface. The children squealed, "Look over there! And there! What *is* that?" Closer investigation revealed we found a clam bar—huge excitement for Midwesterners! We all started digging with our bare hands to capture and study these magnificent sea creatures. It was a simple activity, but I relished the moment because all three of my children were enjoying God's creation at the same time, in the same place.

Meanwhile, I tried to find constructive ways to utilize my time outside our tiny hotel room. My top priority was to make an initial appointment with our new psychiatrist, Dr. Joshi. Dr. Joshi agreed to see us privately as a favor to Dr. Zimmerman. Dr. Joshi was and continues to be one of the most esteemed psychopharmacological researchers in the county; families travel from near and far to receive his help. He specialized in research but also established a private practice. Dr. Joshi's interest was medication management for children with dual diagnoses of bipolar disorder and autistic spectrum disorder.

Since we had been told in the past that Joshua had both of those disorders, Dr. Joshi sounded like a perfect match! Dr. Joshi was very prestigious, and we were willing to sacrifice our time and money. But wow, how these frequent trips burnt holes in our pockets. It cost $200 per thirty minute visit. Of course it was not covered by insurance.

Dr. Joshi was also located in Cambridge so each trip required a difficult choice. I could either drive through Boston in rush-hour traffic, or I could take public transportation (the "T") to its northernmost stop. For each visit I would pick up each child from their respective schools and spend nearly two hours traveling while the kids did homework in the car. Many school nights we did not return home until ten o'clock. It was a brutal schedule, but it was worth it because Dr. Joshi found the perfect medication cocktail. Dr. Joshi continued the Lithium, added Seroquel, and stopped the Tenex. I was amenable to stopping the Tenex since it did nothing more than sedate him.

Eventually the grueling travel during the school week affected the entire family. I searched for another option for a few months and then finally found psychiatric nurse practitioner Mary McDonnell who ran her private practice in Marshfield city twenty minutes away! Mary Ann recently cowrote an excellent book on bipolar disorder with Dr. Janet Wozniak, *Is Your Child Bipolar?: The Definitive Resource on How to Identify, Treat, and Thrive with a Bipolar Child* (Mary Ann McDonnell, 2008). Mary Ann's sessions were a bit less expensive and a lot closer to home. Mary Ann was awesome because she was personable, compassionate, extremely knowledgeable, and responsive to email.

DEPARTMENT OF MENTAL HEALTH

I also pursued services like we had in Pennsylvania. First, I submitted a lengthy application to Massachusetts's Department of Mental Health (DMH) and included copies of all the medical and psychiatric records for their perusal. A week later, DMH called me for an interview to determine Joshua's eligibility. I traveled to Brockton the very next day to re-explain Joshua's life story while my three children fought in the corner.

I did not realize at the time that Joshua's eligibility for DMH services was in serious jeopardy because I presented paperwork that documented two different diagnoses: both bipolar disorder *and* PDD-NOS. The intake committee's responsibility was to determine which diagnosis was most pervasive and thus causing the most limitations. If they determined PDD-NOS was the primary disability then services would be declined and Joshua would only be eligible for services through the Department of Mental Retardation (DMR). If Joshua would have been sent to DMR, and subsequently qualified for their services, assistance would have been menial due to lack of state funding. Praise the Lord the DMH intake committee determined that Joshua's mental health history was the most pervasive, debilitating factor. He qualified!

DMH immediately scheduled a wrap-around intake meeting for the following week. I had absolutely no idea what to expect at this meeting. As I entered the room, twenty compassionate eyes stared intently my way. I couldn't believe ten people were all there to help me and my son. I blinked, then timidly stared wide-eyed at their soft smiles inviting me inside. The best way to describe this meeting was like having Santa Claus ask you what you wanted for Christmas, and then having Santa tell you exactly how his twelve elves were going to get you every present.

The purpose of the meeting was to brainstorm possible programs, resources, and services available to Josh based upon his and my family's unique needs. I was humbled and amazed at their ingenuity and generosity. Although I was a well educated, proactive parent, I was new to the Plymouth area, so the team felt we could benefit from multiple options. They offered to provide me with high intensity wrap services, mentoring, respite, parent support groups, and educational advocacy services.

The purpose of the high intensity "wrap" service was to provide intensive short term assistance for the entire family. For approximately one year, we took advantage of this program. It included a monthly meeting with all of Joshua's service providers. Together we would discuss Joshua's treatment, developmental progress, and future needs.

Josh was also given a therapeutic mentor, who he adored. Each week Miss Carly would take Joshua somewhere special. Miss Carly was an excellent role model who provided counseling and helped boost Joshua's self esteem. Usually they went to Joshua's favorite places, including Friendly's or the arcade. Unfortunately the mentoring services were only meant to be short term, and Miss Carly was required to phase out after six months. The separation was compassionate and deliberately slow, but it was still really difficult on Joshua. It took him much longer than other children to develop trusting relationships, and just when he was growing attached, she had to leave.

Because I was unfamiliar with our new public school system, DMH also provided educational advocacy. We were matched with Mrs. Cunningham through Community Care Services. An educational advocate is someone who represents a child with a disability on behalf of the family by working directly with the school. It was reassuring that Mrs. Cunningham had my back when I dealt with the school. She was definitely an inspiration. She educated me so I could advocate for my son on my own in the future. Witnessing how Mrs. Cunningham helped struggling families became my inspiration. It encouraged me to find employment as the Early Childhood Coordinator for the Wareham School District, and then later to become an independent educational advocate. And the best part about it was that it was all bringing glory to God!

DMH's services seemed endless at that time. They plugged me into a supportive network, the Parent Information Network. Twice a month I would attend meetings with other mothers just like me who were going through the same struggles. The relief I felt at these meetings is indescribable. When I was with these women, I did not have to describe in words the struggles or fears I went through. It was simply understood. It was also an opportunity to share resources on the best hospitals, psychiatrists, and counselors.

DMH placed Joshua into the Therapeutic Aftercare Program (TAP) as well. Every day Joshua would attend their regimented social skills program for two hours. Despite some pitfalls along the way, Joshua successfully completed this program after three years. During this time he worked diligently on social skills, following the rules, sharing feelings, learning to take responsibility for his actions, safety awareness, and ways to demonstrate kindness toward others.

RESPITE

DMH also offered respite services in the western suburbs of Boston. For a few years, Joshua went there on a monthly basis. I would like to pretend that the respite services were for Joshua alone, but the truth is that it provided relief for the entire family. At first I felt terribly guilty sending him away, but quickly I had to admit we all needed a break from each other.

I surmised that Joshua's outlook on respite would depend on my attitude. So with head held high I described weekend camp to Joshua as a place to go where he would get a break from all of Mom's and Dad's rules, while we focused on Alexa and Caleb for a few days. Joshua loved weekend camp, and his behavior was stellar; there was never a behavior incident in over three years!

Respite was positive in every regard; we were able to attend weddings, soccer tournaments, and birthday parties without worry. Joshua trusted that we would always come back in forty-eight hours. For me, however, there were complications with the logistics. The Friday night rush hour traffic and the medication check-in upon arrival were utterly dreadful. I was always anxious to leave quickly so I could battle the traffic once again.

Respite had a disorganized system; every visit they changed the building where we needed to sign in. With each arrival we would go to the building we used the previous visit, only to find that nurses were not available. Then they would send us traipsing across the campus, hauling his pillow and suitcase through cold, blustery nights. When we finally entered the correct building, we had to wait another fifteen minutes for a nurse's arrival. It felt like we were waiting for molasses to flow on a cold winter's day.

I always got excited when the nurse finally arrived; I would eagerly hand her the prescription bottles and the psychiatrist's letter listing the medication so she could start counting pills. One by one by one. I quickly learned I could get back into the wretched traffic quicker if I brought fewer pills in each bottle. Although it expedited the process, I still ran into other roadblocks. There were a few occasions they threatened to not allow him into the program because one of the bottles was not exactly identical to the letter from the psychiatrist.

Since Joshua's medication was being tweaked every few weeks at that time, the writing on the bottle was not explicit enough. Respite wanted a new letter every visit notifying them of changes.

Despite these minor annoyances, respite truly was a gift from above. But it was meant to be temporary. Four years later state budget cuts limited DMH from funding respite. Now it can only be utilized for crisis situations in an effort to prevent an inpatient hospitalization. Yet the Lord was always watching out for us, because soon after respite ended, Dave's parents moved to Plymouth to help out with the kids. It was such a blessing to have them near; they always came to our rescue.

GLASS HALF FULL

In Plymouth, I found new means to maintain positive thoughts. One method I attempted was to create a list of fifteen good things about my day every night before bedtime. I tried to be grateful for my friends, family, health...even the weather.

I needed these lists to keep a balanced perspective on my life. I'm not sure if it was human nature, or just me being vulnerable to frequent negative thoughts, but I was more likely to cling to one negative incident than twenty positive ones. I knew I could only fight this tendency with Scripture, so I plastered Philippians 4:8 in larger letters on my refrigerator so I could see it constantly:

> Finally brothers, whatever is true, whatever is noble, whatever is right, whatever is pure, whatever is lovely, whatever is admirable—if anything is excellent of praiseworthy—think about such things.

It was easier to take care of myself when Joshua was emotionally stable. I found such peace and contentment living by the ocean. I went to the beach constantly; there I felt the closest to God. Hearing the soft crash of the waves and watching the rocks gently tumbling back and forth in sync with the ebb and flow of the water soothed my soul. When I would look out at the landscape and see white billowy clouds stacked against a clear blue sky behind the jetty, all was right with the world. God's creation was my peace, my therapy.

I also read a lot, usually at night until my eye lids become so heavy that Dave would whisper, "Turn the lights off Jamie!" Christian books, self-help books, fiction, and non-fiction alike, I was ready and willing to devour any great book. I also attended a summer Bible Study and went to Celebrate Recovery meetings. Celebrate Recovery is a twelve-step, bible-based program for people with "hurts, habits, or hang-ups."

I made it a priority to share my problems with a few specific people so that I would have a support system in place, and I still had the incredible support system provided by DMH. I scheduled massages, took long bubble baths, and immersed myself in music. I attended a woman's Bible study on Tuesday mornings and committed to the biweekly parent support group.

With my cup half full, I knew without a shadow of a doubt that those difficult times in Pennsylvania were stepping stones toward a better place. Our final destination belonged here along the east coast. I tried to never lose sight of the fact that God gave me my wonderful, unique, and fractured family for a very specific reason; He had great plans for us!

God led us to where community resources and medical care could offer the most help. God placed us in the exact school district that was capable of meeting Joshua's needs. God had it all figured out; nothing happened by accident because He was involved! Sometimes I felt like we were a family of leaves dancing around each other and blowing in the breeze. We were feather-light, and willing to be carried by the wind and settle wherever He chose.

And I felt certain God carried my family to Plymouth. I shared with my dear friend Christi in an email how blessed I felt to live in Plymouth, and how the contentment I felt living here spilled over to my children. I shared with her my efforts to keep Joshy engaged in outdoor activities and be closer to nature. One summer morning I took the kids out for a walk on the beach during low tide. Everyone was thrilled to find sea creatures; Joshy discovered five sand dollars and a starfish. All three children shared their excitement over these treasures.

When we returned home, I encouraged all three children to write. They wrote about everything they were thankful for on the beach that morning, as well as other thanks and praises for who God is and what He's given each of them. Joshy was interested every step of the way, and Alexa and Caleb loved his involvement. Every child wrote their ideas in bright colors on large poster board until it turned into an artwork of rainbow praises. When we ended in prayer, Joshy's words were so vulnerable and heartfelt…it was such a great morning.

KINDERGARTEN...AGAIN

I made the decision when we moved that Joshua would repeat kindergarten. This was another tough decision, but I had to take into consideration his developmental delays and his late summer birthday. I believed repeating kindergarten could provide a great opportunity to reinforce academic pre-readiness skills. Joshua was blessed with a placement in Mrs. Baker's classroom. Mrs. Baker was a lovely teacher with many years of experience; she had a calm, sing-songy voice that soothed the children. She was very patient and tolerant of Joshua's behaviors.

About half way through the school year, I shared my concerns about Joshua's behavior with the school psychologist, and we decided it might help if she conducted a functional behavioral analysis (FBA). As part of the FBA process, the psychologist collected data, comprised a report, and created an IEP with recommendations on how they could help Joshua become more successful in the classroom. The IEP identified positive behaviors to increase, such as raising his hand quietly and monitoring only himself. Target behaviors Joshua needed to decrease included calling out or interrupting when it was not his turn and to diminish his monitoring, bossing, and tattling on others.

Each morning Joshua would decide what reward he would like to earn based on selections from a prize box. Throughout each day Joshua needed to help "froggie" jump to his pond in five leaps using a sticker system. Every thirty minutes Joshua would check in, and if he achieved the targeted behaviors, he would earn a sticker. He needed three stickers out of five to earn the coveted prize. The system was simple yet successful, and we saw improvements within the first week. Later Joshua's behavior plan was modified to include other behaviors such as staying on task and improving his activities of daily living (using tissues, hand washing, zipping his pants, washing his face). This behavior plan worked well within the confines of the classroom, but we never considered a contingency plan for an extraordinary event. The kindergarten spring field trip to the zoo happened to be one of those occasions. The classroom was buzzing with anticipation. Joshua was well cared for with a personal aide, two parent chaperones, and the teacher. He behaved beautifully for the ride down and during his time at the zoo until the ride back home.

Boredom set in during the long ride back to school, so Joshua could not resist the urge to sneak his little hands deep into his backpack full of papers. Marveling at the high winds whipping through the windows, Joshua methodically started to rip his papers into shreds and then release them one at a time into the air. The papers floated everywhere, causing chaos on the bus; all the children were laughing and standing up to catch them. As pieces wafted by the bus driver's field of vision, she yelled to him, "Knock it off!" But the negative attention from the children only fueled the fire as Joshua continued to launch pieces of paper.

Imagine Joshua's dismay when he was sent straight to the principal's office. He truly didn't know what was so wrong with his little experiment. Not only did he struggle with personal accountability, but his impulsivity also prevented him for considering the consequences of his actions. At home that night, I reminded him of the importance of listening to authority and explained how his behavior jeopardized everyone's safety. But deep inside I knew my little sensory seeker had experienced something spectacular. With the windows open and air rushing all around, he was infatuated with the new sensation on his skin and the visual display of paper wafting through the air.

HEATBREAK

T he last week of the school year, I received an unexpected phone call from Mrs. Baker. She informed me that Joshua had been bullying other children relentlessly, and that parents were calling the school because naturally, they were upset. I was horrified to learn that one parent even requested her daughter *not* be in the same classroom as Joshua the following year.

It was easiest to seethe with anger first. Anxious thoughts swirled through my head, *Why didn't Mrs. Baker tell me about Joshua's behavior sooner? How could she let the situation escalate without communicating with me until now.* But very quickly my feelings switched to guilt. *How could I be so blind to what is happening with my son? Haven't I taught him about gentleness, kindness, and compassion? How could I overlook the possibility that he could end up a perpetrator himself?* Joshy's behavior was contrary to everything we believed in or taught him. We were teaching him to love others! We were teaching him to have gentle hands! We were teaching kind words! We were teaching him empathy and faith in Jesus! *Lord, please show me where we gone wrong!* I prayed. I couldn't decide whether Joshy's behavior was related to our weaknesses in parenting, was of his free will, or was uncontrolled due to his disabilities.

It is one thing to know that your child has struggles, but when you realize that even the strangers around you are aware, it causes heartbreak. When they do not want your child to play with their child, it stings. And when they talk behind your back, it kills. My heart was breaking again at the realization that my son was on his way to becoming an outcast because of his eccentric and unsafe behaviors. That summer I reinforced to

Joshua the perils of bullying, and I equipped him with ways to treat others with gentleness and kindness.

That summer I thought my training had equipped Joshua to navigate relationships better, so when the bus came to pick him for Camp Clark each day, I had minimal concern. But one day at camp, the activity Joshua was participating in was cut short because it was time to come home. Reluctantly he got on the bus and unbeknownst to the driver, he was drowning in agitation and anger in the back seat. Joshua never said a word.

On the thirty minute journey home, the driver thought she heard the smaller child next to Joshua whimpering in the back seat, but she was not suspicious as she looked in her rearview mirror. This little child was strapped into his car seat; he was much younger, severely disabled, and nonverbal. Very quietly Joshua stewed in his anger until he couldn't take it any longer. To cope, Joshua started embedding his fingernails deeply into the skin on the little boy's legs. Repeatedly. When the bus arrived and I helped Joshua out of the car, I saw the blood running everywhere on the little boys legs. I slowly put the pieces of the puzzle together and learned that Joshua hurt this little guy. My heart sank, I was devastated.

I yanked Joshua into the house and immediately started crying and screaming at him. I sobbed for the helpless child in the van. He was also bawling, begging for forgiveness. I could not even interact with him I was so ashamed and disappointed in his behavior. I never imagined he would do something so ugly to another human being. I felt like I was going to throw up. I could not excuse this behavior; I could not bear to look at him. He was sent to his room for a few hours. I knew it wasn't the best solution, but I had to find a short term separation for us because I knew I was going to blow if he opened his mouth. It was a dark day. I learned that no matter how much we prepared or taught Joshua for life, certain things were simply out of our control.

After consulting with Dave, we worked with Joshua diligently to reinforce better ways to handle his anger. I also called the mother of the little boy and offered my sincerest apologies. Thankfully she was merciful and gracious about the entire encounter and offered her forgiveness for Joshua's behavior. Joshua also apologized to the mother and the little boy, as well as wrote him a letter describing his regret. This letter was his repentance because handwriting was not only difficult but also very painful for his fingers.

BEHAVIOR PLANS

With a heightened sense of awareness regarding car behavior, I implemented a new behavior system during car rides for all the children. I hoped that my plan would reduce the chaos and fighting during travel. I laminated a sheet titled "Dollar Rewards" and photocopied fake dollar bills to hand out as incentives. For every car trip the kids had an opportunity to earn dollar bills by following simple rules. The first thing I needed was three basic rules.

1. (one) Keep your hands to yourself.
2. (two) Mind your own business.

   a. No tattling
   b. No interrupting
   c. No fighting

3. (three) Quiet voices when driver is speaking.

   1. On telephone
   2. Ordering food at drive thru
   3. At bank or pharmacy drive thru

The second requirement was a reward system.

10 Dollars:

   1. (one) Your choice of DVD during next car ride.
   2. (two) Special snack of choice.
   3. (three) Stay up 30 minutes later at bedtime.

20 Dollars:

1. (one) Earn $2.00 cash.
2. (two) Special time with parent of choice for one hour.
3. (three) Pick DVD rental for popcorn movie night.

30 Dollars:

1. (one) Sleep in mom and dad's room on the weekend.
2. (two) Select school snacks for an entire week.
3. (three) No chores for two weekdays.

40 Dollars:

1. (one) Choose a friend for a sleepover.
2. (two) Special time with parent of choice for two hours.
3. (three) Choose a friend for a play date.

Finally, the third requirement described the consequences each car ride.

Strike 1:   Warning.
Strike 2:   1 dollar taken away.
Strike 3:   2 dollars taken away.
Strike 4:   3 dollars taken away plus 30 minute time out.

Although the system worked beautifully, I admit it was difficult to be consistent after a few months passed. Eventually we faded out the protocols when their behaviors improved and so many other areas needed to be addressed with Joshua. Another tactic I implemented was a stoplight behavior system for Joshua and Caleb one summer. First, I described the different color levels.

Green:

1. (one) I was safe.
2. (two) I used my quiet voice.
3. (three) I handled transitions well (no whining, tantrums, or refusals).

Yellow:

1. (one) I was safe but.....
2. (two) I shouted out.
3. (three) I handled transitions poorly.

Red:

1. (one) I was unsafe (hitting, kicking, pushing, spitting, threatening, throwing objects, running away, destroying property).
2. (two) I was already on yellow and continued to shout or handle transition poorly.

There were two check-ins for their levels, at lunch and dinner, and based on behavior they would move an icon to the accurate level. Again, there were rewards and consequences based on the level they earned. The system became an excellent way to help Joshua evaluate himself and pay closer attention to his behavior.

MEDICAL MYSTERY NUMBER THREE

One thing I've never understood about New England's public school system is the notorious, weeklong winter break scheduled every February. The winter break is torturous for parents because the children come home and have nothing to do except stare out the window at the crummy weather. Then the poor kids do not get out of school for summer break until late in June, when instead they should be enjoying the sunshine at the beach.

This was our first winter break on the east coast, and I knew the thrill of sledding would only last a few days, so I decided to entertain them with a road trip. I dropped off Joshua at his grandparents' house in Connecticut, and then I traveled out to Pennsylvania and New Jersey with Alexa and Caleb. After a few days, Dave picked up Joshua from his parent's house, and together they returned to Plymouth hoping for some quality father-son time.

While I was visiting with my favorite cousin Julie out in New Jersey, Dave called to tell me Joshua was ill again. He said Joshua had hives and a low grade fever while he was at his grandparents' house and by the time they returned to Plymouth, Joshua was having increased joint pain and swelling—again. The pain was so intense that he could barely walk or move again.

Dave took him to Jordan Hospital's Emergency Room, which proved only an effort of futility; they had no clue what was causing these symptoms. Disbelief compounded our fear as we realized that this was the *third* time we had dealt with this mysterious malady! I rushed home from New Jersey so we could take Joshua to Mass General's Emergency Room. But even the best doctors at Mass General could not pinpoint the cause. Perplexed, they arranged for him to see their top pediatric rheumatologist the next day. Joshua presented with swollen eyes, swollen knees, redness, tenderness, and scattered rashes. He could not raise his shoulders or bear weight. Dr. Wheeler, the rheumatologist, thoroughly examined Joshua, obtained a blood sample, then went home to research and contemplate the symptoms. Dr. Wheeler later confided in me that he lost sleep over this case. We anticipated a diagnosis such as juvenile arthritis or an auto immune disease, but everything came back negative. Meanwhile, the pain and swelling mysteriously subsided within three days.

The next day Dr. Wheeler called me. His best guess was that Joshua may have had an allergic reaction to penicillin, because the hives appeared on the ninth day of a ten day prescription of penicillin (previously prescribed for an ear infection.) Dr. Wheeler prescribed Joshua naproxen (for swelling) and Benadryl (an antihistamine), all which I could have gotten from the local doctor. Needless time, money, and emotion were wasted. *This trip to the doctor has been a total nuisance today! We still don't have any answers!* I fumed.

As I watched my little boy inexplicably suffer, I prayed 2 Corinthians 12:9 over him:

> But he said to me, "My grace is sufficient for you, for my power is made perfect in weakness." Therefore I will boast all the more gladly about my weaknesses, so that Christ's power may rest on me. This beautiful verse gave me hope.

THE INVESTIGATION

The summer when Joshua turned seven was very difficult. My mother always loved visiting with her grandchildren, so she came for a wonderful, two-week visit that July. Joshua was emotionally unstable, so my mother's support helped immensely.

One afternoon I was determined to take everybody to the beach to force them to have fun. As we drove to the beach, Joshua abruptly fixated upon his desire for some ice cream. He obsessed about going to Friendly's rather than the ocean. He was relentless and persistent with his wishes, but I had to tell him no because we were almost to the beach.

When Joshua realized he was not going to Friendly's, he became belligerent and started kicking seats and screaming. I wasn't sure how to respond with my mother and kids in the car; I wanted to keep the peace. I wondered if I should ignore Joshua's temper trantrum or turn the car around and head home as a consequence for his behavior. But consequences for Joshua often became everyone else's consequence as well; the kids and I missed out on many activities over the years (e.g. beach days) because Joshua couldn't handle the stress of a new activity. I dreaded acknowledging his misbehavior, yet I knew I had to respond to his unacceptable behavior. With a big sigh, I turned the car around to take my disappointed kids home as quickly as possible.

Since Joshua was still agitated, I sent him to his room to cool off. This provided me a break as well. I was embarrassed and frustrated by his behavior; I couldn't escape these constant meltdowns! Although my mother was trying to reassure me that things were going to get better, I could hear Joshua upstairs trashing his bedroom, throwing things at the walls. My anger was swelling inside as I listened to him destroy our property. Finally when I could take no more, I marched up the stairs to enter his room.

As I approached his bedroom door, a plastic toy was lying on the floor of the hallway that belonged in his room. Adrenaline flowing through my veins, I picked up the toy, swung open the door, and launched it. It happened in an instant, in anger I aimlessly threw the toy into his bedroom without looking. I screamed, "Be quiet!" then slammed the door shut.

Then, I stood back, frozen in horror at what had just occurred. There was no thinking involved, only raw emotion and thoughtless reflex. I opened the door again to rush to his side and see the damage. Toys were broken, the walls were marked, and all the clothes were thrown out of drawers. Then I looked at him. Aghast, I saw minor swelling and some bruising starting to appear near his right temple. Apparently my blind throw grazed Joshua's right temple/eye and now he was howling.

The incident could have been a careless accident on any given day when I toss toys into their room, but this was different. I threw it in anger. I comforted his tears with kisses and ice as we wept together. I had never felt so low. I wondered what happened to me and who I had become. I couldn't comprehend how I was so calm and collected earlier, only to have thrown that toy in anger and hurt my son. I felt like a monster. *How could I have lost sight of James 1:19 (*KJV*) that commands me to be swift to hear, slow to speak, and slow to wrath?* I desperately prayed.

Nobody could have made me feel worse than I already did. I cried out to God that I didn't deserve anything. Comfort, love, happiness, I was not worthy. I hated myself and was filled with anguish and remorse. Joshua and I finally calmed down and together we prayed; I asked the Lord for forgiveness while we clung tight to the each other. That night I realized I felt exactly how Joshua must feel about himself after every single outburst. Wow. To live with that lack of control and then to experience that subsequent remorse must be indescribable.

The next morning Joshua went to Camp Clark with a bruise on his temple. He left the house showering me with hugs and kisses, but the first thing he did at camp was tell Kay, the TAP case manger, "My mommy hit me last night." Kay reluctantly called me to inquire about the incident, because we had a great relationship and she knew I was very attentive and gentle with Joshua.

I had a baseball-sized pit in my stomach while I explained the altercation. Because I worked in the social services field, I knew she was a mandated reporter and had to file a report with the Department of Child & Family (DCF). I was sick to my stomach. I had just accepted my new position in the Wareham Public Schools as the Early Childhood Coordinator, and an accusation such as this could jeopardize my career and, worse yet, my family.

When Joshua returned home and we discussed the impending investigation and its ramifications, he was filled with dread at the thought that he would be taken away from his parents. With such limited expressive communication skills, he could not articulate the circumstances or that the incident was an accident. But the wheels were now in motion and protocols needed to be followed. The following week, Joshua tried to put on a brave face while a kind gentleman from DCF came to the home to interview us. The investigation was immediately dropped, but I still never forgave myself.

Camp Clark Explosion

I was ecstatic about my new job as the Early Childhood Coordinator for the Wareham Public School District. I embraced my new responsibilities which included managing special education services and programming for preschool students. But back at home, the anxiety produced by DCF's investigation became the catalyst for another inpatient psychiatric hospitalization. Joshua was still attending Camp Clark, but he was markedly agitated and emotional over small stressors or demands placed upon him. One unsuspecting day rather than taking the bus home from camp, I arrived near the end of the day to pick up Joshua for his psychiatrist appointment. I parked the car then made the long walk down into the courtyard surrounded by three buildings and a gorgeous lake.

I found Joshua down by the water just finishing swim time.

"Hi sweetie! Guess what? It's time to go see Mary Ann like we talked about this morning. Let's go honey!"

Joshua grumbled, kicked stones, and stalled his departure as he ran over to the bubbler.

"Joshua, we really need to leave quickly for your appointment," I reminded him.

But Joshua was in no mood to be told what to do. Suddenly he started running aimlessly around the courtyard screaming. After Kay and I chased him around the courtyard for a few minutes, we finally caught him. I just couldn't understand how this escalated. I reminded him that morning that I would be picking him up early, and I knew how much he loved going to the doctor and getting undivided attention. I agonized over why he might be freaking out

Impulsively, Joshua picked up stones and started throwing and kicking them toward innocent bystanders. Naturally, a large crowd started to gather, and I thought I was going to break into tiny pieces inside while watching Joshua make such a spectacle of himself. Because Joshua was clearly demonstrating unsafe behavior, we finagled him into the nearest vacant building. Kay manipulated his body into a non-invasive basket hold, but Joshua's adrenaline was so revved that the two of us could barely keep him from lashing out. Kay was scratched and punched many times while I sat on the periphery, helplessly crying.

We all agreed that Joshua needed to be transported to Jordan Hospital for a crisis evaluation. They wanted to call an ambulance but I refused; I just could not envision a noisy ambulance making its way down into this courtyard while peers stared and snickered under their breath. I finally convinced the staff to agree to let me personally transport him. I ran to my vehicle and slowly drove it into the courtyard where no car was ever meant to travel. When Joshua finally calmed down, he had no recollection of the incident. When we explained what happened, he was absolutely beside himself. Remorseful, repentant, and deflated, Joshua knew he needed what we termed help.

Joshy and I waited for six hours while the social worker completed a thorough intake and began the referral process for an inpatient hospital stay with our insurance company. Joshy lied on a narrow stretcher in the hallway amidst the hustle and bustle of life threatening emergencies. Mercifully they eventually moved him into a small private room with a 1980's TV and some Sponge Bob Squarepants VHS tapes. When it was finally time to leave we were transported via ambulance. I insisted I go with Joshy in the back of the ambulance to ameliorate his fears....and mine. The entire process did not seem to be getting any easier with experience.

WESTWOOD LODGE

We accepted an expedited inpatient psychiatric placement at Westwood Lodge Hospital in the western suburbs of Boston. We didn't know anything about the program, except that our insurance company agreed to cover his stay. Upon arrival we quickly learned that Westwood Lodge offered a variety of acute psychiatric services for children and adolescents in emotional crisis.

Lord, how do I cope with Joshua being in the hospital again? Honestly, it feels like I'm on vacation, but to feel this way seems vicious and cruel. My other children need me, Lord. Alexa and Caleb get pushed aside because I'm catering to Joshua's needs. I just don't know how to juggle this anymore. How many more hats do you want me to wear? Every night I fall in bed utterly exhausted. I stink at parenting. It's hard to forgive myself when I fall short in my parenting role.

Help me never to forget to pray every night the meditation of the heart that I whisper over Joshua, "Lord, give Joshua peace of mind, peace of heart, and peace of soul." But when I put my hands on his sweet smelling skin, (a combination of lollipops, toothpaste, and his special blankie), I am still able to cherish that single, quiet moment every evening. I try to remember that You gave me this child for a reason. I trust in You. I know You have great plans for the both of us. You have it all figured out. With you, nothing is an accident.

Unfortunately, Joshua's experience at Westwood proved to be highly disappointing. His case manager was impersonal and unorganized, and I found myself coordinating more resources and meetings on Joshua's behalf than she did. Joshua remained in acute stabilization for five days. After that they recommended a less intensive, small group, step-down program for another week. We were skeptical of his success in a small group because it required a high level of social skills and sustained attention, both of which were difficult for Joshua. We also explained our concerns about the daily commute to the program, but they convinced us the hassle and expense was worth it because they could do wonders.

Contrary to Westwood's promise, Joshua's participation in their program validated our original concern that it was an inappropriate placement. His discharge summary stated, "Joshua has difficulty staying on task, difficulty focusing, needs limits defined, has no sense of boundaries, and has poor social interactions. Furthermore, Joshua's presentation qualifies a diagnosis of ADHD, oppositional-defiant disorder (a type of personality disorder), and Asperger's Disorder (AS)."

Can there possibly be two more diagnoses? How dare these people who knew my son for only a week tell me that he has a personality disorder? Who do they think they are trying to label my son at the tender age of eight? I thought. I was certain my son had a mood imbalance, not a personality defect. When his emotions were regulated, there was never any opposition to authority. They did not see Joshua's gentle heart; they did not know he truly wanted to please others, to love and be loved.

The team wrote, "Given Joshua's disability of Asperger's, this program could not help him. He lacked the insight and communication skills required to make progress in this program." I felt coerced into the suggestion, he gained nothing from the experience, and then they trampled all over us with their callous remarks attached to a non-existent future treatment plan.

Joshua left Westwood with an increase in his seroquel prescription 300 mg, lithium 150 mg, and tenex 1mg. The tenex was their "hail Mary" attempt at curbing the hyperactivity and impulsivity. I told them it didn't work when he was younger, but they didn't believe me. When Joshua's stay at Westwood was nearing its end, I reached out to my faithful prayer warriors again.

Dear Prayer Warriors,

We had a productive meeting at the hospital on Friday. We know the direction things are heading at this point. Joshua is going to be discharged on Monday at 4:30 p.m. Dave will be there to pick him up. There are three weeks of summer left before school begins out here.

Westwood has recommended Joshua go to a step-down program during this time to ease his transition back into the "real world." Our insurance has agreed to pay for this at least for the first week, so we are going to give it a whirl. This sounds best for Joshua, although the sacrifice is for us to drive him up there through Boston traffic daily at 9:30 and 2:30. DMH has agreed to reimburse us for transportation costs, which will help immensely. I don't know how we will get through the commuting logistics, but Dave's employer is flexible, and we will plow through it.

If this step-down program does not work, then Joshua can go to our dear friends' house (George and Janet Shipp) before school starts back up. There he can play with their grandsons. Joshua loves it at their house, so it's a good second alternative.

In the meanwhile, we are in the process of securing a therapist, and I am requesting an emergency TE a.m. meeting with the public schools. There will likely be about ten people there, including the out of district liaison that specializes in placing kids like Joshua in other programs at the school district's expense. DMH has given us an educational advocate who will help us "fight" for these services if we have to. This is free—big praise for that! I will walk into the meeting with recommendations from two psychiatrists that it is in Joshua's best interest to attend a therapeutic program that can provide the structure he needs to thrive. I am also requesting occupational therapy and physical therapy evaluations as well as looking for an outside neuropsychological evaluation. It is so much!

On the home front, Dave and I are reevaluating everything we need to do (and change) within our family so we can all coexist better. We need to learn that we cannot push him and "normalize" him into things. We still have to provide a daily schedule to help him self-regulate. This seems like a massive undertaking. Please pray for our safety as we commute him back and forth the next few weeks, and pray for continuity and strength as we bring our family back together. Pray that we would not become overwhelmed and for Joshua to have peace. Peace of heart, mind, and soul. Thank you prayer warriors for your love and concern. Jamie

ASPERGER'S DISORDER?

As disappointed as I was with Westwood, I knew I still had a responsibility to educate myself on Joshua's new diagnosis of Asperger's disorder. Asperger's disorder is one of five specific pervasive developmental disorders listed. I absorbed new information through web searches and my trusty DSM-IV.

> Asperger's is characterized by a qualitative impairment in social interaction, as manifested by at least two of the following:
>
> 1. (one) Impairment of nonverbal behaviors (eyes contact, facial expression, gestures).
> 2. (two) Lack of social emotional reciprocity.
> 3. (three) Failure to develop peer relationships appropriate to age development.
> 4. (four) Lack of spontaneous seeking to share enjoyment, entertainment, or interests with others.
>
> Asperger's is also characterized by restricted, repetitive, and stereotyped patterns of behavior, interests, and activities, as manifested by at least one of the following:
>
> 1. (one) Inflexible adherence to nonfunctional routines or rituals.
> 2. (two) Stereotyped and repetitive motor mannerisms (i.e. Hand flapping, twisting, pacing, toe walking) and persistent preoccupation with objects rather than people (i.e. Watching ceiling fans or the pendulum on a clock swinging rhythmically.)

JAMIE BIERUT

Furthermore, there must be impairment in social, occupational, or other important areas of functioning. Criteria must not be met for another pervasive developmental disorder or schizophrenia, and there must not be a clinically significant delay in cognitive development or age-appropriate self-help skills, adaptive behavior, and curiosity about the environment. People with Asperger's Disorder may also be very good at basic communication skills, but they often struggle with imagination, organizational skills, literal interpretations, nonverbal cues (gestures, body language), self expression, initiating conversation, and eye contact. Many may also have sensory processing disorders (American Psychiatric Association, 2000).

With the criteria laid out before me in black and white, I studied the list over and over. Despite this new diagnosis I could not believe it. Yes, Joshua had delayed nonverbal behaviors such as limited eye contact and awkward facial gestures. He did miss social cues and have social awkwardness's. Yes, Joshua desperately needed consistent routines and rituals because his adaptive skills were poor. Yes, he was not interested in sharing other's interests if they did not benefit him in some way. And yes, he did not have the skills necessary to obtain and maintain relationships with peers.

But on the contrary, Joshua was highly attuned to other people's emotional states and responded with compassion and empathy from a very early age. He was also willing to seek and share mutual enjoyment with others, and he never demonstrated repetitive movements such as hand flapping. And unlike many children with Asperger's disorder, Joshua had significant delays with communication, adaptive behaviors, and self help skills. I may not have been a psychiatrist, but

184

these factors were plenty enough to convince me not to label my son with Asperger's disorder. I just wish I knew what the missing puzzle piece was and if there was truly one diagnosis that described Josh.

A Mother Prays for Mercy

After taking these diagnostic criteria into consideration, I agreed that many of Joshua's traits matched. Yet something deep inside of me still knew there was a missing piece. As I studied Matthew 15:21-28 many questions resurfaced in regard to spiritual warfare and healing. Scripture reads:

> Jesus left that place and went off to the territory near the cities of Tyre and Sidon. A Canaanite woman who lived in that region came to him.
>
> "Son of David!" she cried out. "Have mercy on me, sir! My daughter has a demon and is in a terrible condition."
>
> But Jesus did not say a word to her. His disciples came to him and egged him, "Send her away! She is following us and making all this noise!"
>
> Then Jesus replied, "I have been sent only to the lost sheep of the people of Israel."
>
> At this the woman came and fell at his feet. "Help me, sir!" she said.
>
> Jesus answered, "It isn't right to take the children's food and throw it to the dogs."
>
> "That's true, sir," she answered; "but even the dogs eat the leftovers that fall from their masters' table."
>
> So Jesus answered her, "You are a woman of great faith! What you want will be done for you." And at that very moment her daughter was healed."

I felt very confused and unsettled after pouring over these verses, so I reached out to my pastor for clarity.

Dear Pastor,

I tried to catch you after second service, but was unsuccessful. The message today has stirred within me a few questions that maybe you could help me process. Okay, this topic is most interesting to me because of Joshua. Joshua started hearing voices when he was only four years old. They tormented him. I actually took Joshua to a healing ministry in Georgia because he seemed so vulnerable to spiritual warfare. After this trip to the healing ministry, he never heard voices again! Still, much sickness and turmoil remains. How do I truly discern a worldly problem versus a spiritual predicament? I feel like I am this woman in Matthew, begging Jesus again to her child. This is what I don't understand:

You mentioned there are tests we all will endure throughout our lives—faith, love, forgiveness, etc. You said that Jesus rewarded this woman for her faith and thus healed her child. So I am wondering, how could I have possibly not passed God's faith test? If I didn't believe God could control everything and heal my son, I never would have taken him to a healing ministry. What if I have enough faith, but He still doesn't answer my prayer for the child I love? Do you have to pass both tests—faith *and* love? What if I don't love Joshua enough the way God made him? If I did, then maybe, just maybe He would heal him completely? I don't know. I just have difficulty making sense of this pain—mine and Joshua's—in the midst of God's promises.

Dear Jamie,

Be careful about connecting "great faith" with Jesus's decision to heal that woman's daughter. When Jesus praised her, he clearly declared that what he had seen was an example of great faith, but nowhere did he imply that only when someone exhibits great amounts of faith will His power be available. That passage tells us that the unnamed woman claimed her daughter had a demon. Jesus didn't claim that or even address the demon issue. He simple told her that he was impressed with her faith and that her daughter was healed. He didn't even imply that her faith had healed her daughter.

It is possible that some maladies that secular psychologists and psychiatrists treat chemically are really spiritual issues. But many of the issues are also bio-chemical in nature. So on one hand, never rule out what the doctors say, but on the other hand, never rule out the miraculous! Sometimes God only unleashes His miraculous power when we pray.

Finally, God doesn't directly *cause* many of the bad things that we deal with in life, but there is no doubt in my mind that he *uses* these things to test us. Testing has a positive and negative side. From the positive, God wants to stretch us and to prove the strength and character He is building within us. Negatively, some tests push us to the limits simply because we live in a broken world. To a certain degree, we all deal with some level of suffering, brokenness, sickness, and pain. It is part of this world. One thing I would greatly caution you again is ever giving way to the temptation to think that you or your actions are responsible for Joshua's condition. Whatever Joshua is dealing with is not a reflection of your quality of faith. Satan uses stuff like that to guilt-trip and immobilizes believers. Stay strong!

THE OUTER BANKS

My stress level was at an astronomical high that summer. Luckily I knew it was critical to take care of myself so I could be who God made me to be. Outside of the obvious methods such as reading my Bible, surrounding myself with positive people, attending church. I placed Celebrate Recovery and family vacations as my top priorities. Celebrate Recovery is a Bible-based 12 step recovery ministry for people with "hurts, habits, or hang-ups." This includes all addictions, codependency, unhealthy behaviors, and emotional struggles. I sought refuge from the fellowship and guidance of the people attending the program.

I also jumped at the opportunity for a family vacation. Dave readily agreed, but this was yet another one of the many tough decisions we faced because Joshua was on an emotional slippery slope.

We agonized over this decision for days, finally agreeing that if Dave's parents would take him for the week, then we would go. Something in my gut told me we were delaying an inevitable re-hospitalization, yet we forged ahead. At least it was a comfort knowing Joshua could not wait to spend time with Grammy and Grampy. Although the trip to the Outer Banks that fall was amazing, Joshua was never far from my heart or mind. I mourned that Joshua was missing out on family memories.

I struggled to accept that Joshua was too sick to have the same experiences we did. He was content within the world we provided him. For Joshua, less was more. He needed the comfort provided by predictable people and routines. I left two pages of instructions for his grandparents before we left, including emergency numbers, behavior management techniques, and a detailed daily schedule. They embraced the challenge they knew they were headed for, and Joshua remained in their wonderful care.

While we were gone, Dave's mother took excellent notes. The first day Joshua awoke with pupils dilated, fingers constantly snapping, and opening and closing his hands. Most mornings he awoke with anxiety and defiance. He would often kick, hit, scream, and swear. He could not be alone for a single minute because every choice he made was inappropriate or dangerous. He could not settle in and seemed uncomfortable in his own skin. As Joshua described it, he felt "jumpy, jumpy."

Joshua was spiraling downward fast. His body would remain restless and agitated until Grampy would gently lie on him which provided deep pressure to calm him down. As deeply as Joshua loved his Grammy and wanted her near, one day in a fit of rage, he started shooting Nerf darts, swearing, and kicking her. He needed constant supervision to redirect his behavior from poking, kicking, and throwing objects. During another incident Joshua dashed out the back door, running aimlessly into the woods. Thankfully, Joshua was no match to Grampy's speed and agility; Grampy quickly caught up and tackled him to the ground into the safety of his arms.

Joshua regressed that week. He lost the skills required to care for himself and his coordination was off kilter. He couldn't even sit up straight. He would just tilt sideways. Joshua would fall over from a *sitting* position. Furthermore, his new medication seemed to make him very sleepy in the morning. With eyes drooping, he stared through the television with a vacant glaze.

Joshua clung to his personal schedule and loved his chewing gum. One night during his bedtime routine, Grammy reluctantly doled out multiple warnings for misbehavior. When the warnings did not work, with reticence she withheld his gum for the rest of the evening. When Joshua realized that he was being punished by his own grandmother who loved him to pieces and spoiled him rotten, he could not stop crying. Grammy described his grief and sorrow as if his heart was breaking.

When we returned from the Outer Banks and heard the details of Joshua's emotional status, Dave and I realized that it was critical to get stabilized before he could go to school.

BATMAN AND ROBIN

Our first weekend back in Plymouth, Dave and I went on a date with other couples from Bible study. Getting a babysitter was nearly impossible; we had no family nearby, and babysitters for special needs children were a dime a dozen. Luckily, we found a thirteen-year-old babysitter who had successfully watched all three children in the past without incident.

Dave and I could barely contain our excitement that evening. We were meeting our friends for a sunset cruise through Plymouth Harbor on the Pilgrim Belle. Prior to the cruise, we enjoyed a romantic meal alone by the water. After the meal when we journeyed toward the pier to board the Pilgrim Belle, my phone started ringing. It was the babysitter, and she was sobbing hysterically; I could hear the kids screaming in the background as well. Adrenaline started pumping. I instinctively knew something was wrong.

I heard some jumbled phrases, "Josh ran away," and, "he is throwing huge rocks at us." I told her I would call 911, and we would race back home to find Joshua. On a good day, Joshua was barely aware of his surroundings and could easily get hit by a car; he had no safety awareness. But on a *bad* day? I couldn't even fathom the danger he could be in. If Joshua ran frantically into the road without looking, he would be flattened by a car. As we dashed to our car I thanked the Lord that we did not set sail before we received our babysitter's phone call. We would have been helpless out on the water if the call came any later.

Dave drove home tripling the speed limit. Although we made it home in less than ten minutes the police and ambulance won the race. I cringed as I saw our neighbors to the left and right standing outside their homes watching the drama unfold. I ran up to the house where the children were crying. I didn't know where to turn first. Flustered, I wondered whether to tend to my traumatized babysitter and two children, or to help search for Joshua.

I listened while the three of them explained what happened. Apparently they were all playing dress up in the basement when Joshua got upset with his siblings. Despite the babysitter's attempts at calming him, Joshua's anger escalated until he combusted. He ran upstairs and ransacked the bathroom. Joshua locked himself in there and swiped everything out of the cabinets and off the shelves. Plastics and glass were shattered and the other children were terrified.

The babysitter tried to talk to Joshua from outside the bathroom door, but she could not calm him down enough to listen. Suddenly he opened the door, shoved everyone aside, and tore out the front door of the house. They all chased Joshua and begged for him to return, but at this point, Joshua knew he crossed the line; he was scared of being in trouble for his behavior. Next, Joshua started throwing large rocks at them to keep them at a distance. Finally, he turned and ran away, dashing through the neighbor's yards.

Bless her heart, the poor babysitter was beside herself. She didn't know what to do! On one hand, she could not let him run far away, yet on the other, she could not leave the other two alone back at the house hysterical. That's when she called me.

With the babysitter's mother on the way, I flew into the back yard and heard the policeman telling Dave that they spotted Joshua in the woods about fifty yards away crouched behind a boulder amongst the thick trees. Tentatively, quietly, I approached. I whispered, "Joshy, it's me, Mommy. It's okay. You can come out to me. You are safe. I won't let anybody hurt you. I love you no matter what." Slowly Joshua emerged and behold, there before me stood a broken, terrified, sobbing little boy dressed in a Batman and Robin costume. Dirt meshed with tears stained his cheeks as he jumped into my arms. He was shaking and sobbing. He apologized profusely about being "a very bad boy." His pleading eyes told me all I needed to know. He was safe for tonight, but he was suffering inside. That night as Dave and I scratched our heads, we pleaded with God to give us some answers. He was swift to answer at the TAP program the following day:

> A humble prayer request to our friends:
>
> Joshua was transported via ambulance to the hospital tonight around five thirty after assaultive and aggressive behavior at the TAP program. It was triggered by a seemingly insignificant event. Apparently he was not allowed to have a piece of candy until he earned the privilege. He did not want to earn the candy, so instead he became assaultive and kicked the program manager.
>
> As Joshua proceeded to destroy the sensory room, the staff called 911. They wanted to transport him via ambulance by himself. I shuddered at how terrifying this would be for a seven-year-old; there was no way he was riding up there alone. I pleaded with them to give me twenty minutes to get there. Hastily I gathered Alexa and Caleb's overnight bags and sent them to the Shipp's house for the evening.
>
> Next, I then raced to the TAP program across town. I scooped up my weeping little boy and held him the entire ambulance ride. This time Dave was prepared to spend the night in the emergency room while we waited for a bed at a better hospital. We were placed on the wait list for Franciscan Children's Hospital.
>
> We were comforted in our belief that everything escalated again because only God knows what Joshua

truly needs. In some bizarre way, this crisis will help Joshua receive additional support and proper medication, so we had to trust the process. Our hearts sense that Joshua's needs far beyond our abilities.

In the meanwhile, I humbly request you pray for the following needs. Pray for our family as we do not feel we can continue to exist with all this dysfunction. Pray we get accomplished everything God wants us to and that we have the discernment needed to put aside responsibilities that are not critical right now. Pray that Dave and I can juggle our work responsibilities in the middle of this crisis. Pray I can find an attorney or advocate who can guide me through this process. Pray for Alexa and Caleb: Alexa prematurely steps up her mothering and nurturing in my absence, and Caleb is very scared and misses his brother terribly.

We love you all! Jamie

ANNA JAQUES

The placement for Franciscan never came, and we had to settle for Anna Jaques, a private hospital near the northern border of Massachusetts. I was cynical about this new hospital because nothing was accomplished at Westwood Lodge. Thankfully, Anna Jaques proved us wrong. They provided better communication and a high quality of care for their patients.

Anna Jaques was instrumental in two ways. The first discovery was that Joshua's lithium level was at a .69, which was at the low end of the therapeutic range. This level was very low for Joshua; the level at which he maintained mood stabilization was 1.0. The doctor ordered an increase to his lithium dosage. Joshua remained in their hospital for about seven days until his lithium level increased.

The second advantage of Anna Jaques was how they focused on the importance of an appropriate classroom placement for Joshua. I was informed Joshua's best chances for academic and social success would be in a therapeutic classroom. It was refreshing that the doctors were not interested in coming up with more labels to describe Joshua; they were more interested in helping him function in this great big world. I was instructed to request an Emergency TE a.m. meeting with the public schools before Joshua was released from the hospital.

School Matters

To: Plymouth School District

RE: Emergency TE a.m. Meeting for Joshua Bierut

Today Joshua is being released from another psychiatric inpatient stabilization unit at Anna Jaques. Joshua's team of caregivers has brought to my attention that I need to request this meeting to discuss Joshua's well being and educational needs.

Unfortunately, since the start of the summer, Joshua's mental health condition and behavior have declined significantly, despite being involved in a therapeutic summer camp program offered through TAP. Joshua continues to demand more and more emotional and developmental resources than we originally considered.

I would appreciate an IEP meeting to be scheduled this week to discuss accommodations, extended summer services, and placement options. Furthermore, I will be providing documentation from two psychiatrists recommending a therapeutic school placement.

I am also requesting a PT and OT evaluation. He continues to demonstrate delays in his activities of daily living and ability to care for himself. He also struggles with gross motor and fine motor skills. Thank you so much for your support and care for my child! I look forward to talking with you soon when you choose a date for this meeting.

Sincerely, Jamie Bierut

I also wrote a second letter with the help and approval of Josh's psychiatrist Dr. Joshi. We described Josh's current psychiatric diagnoses, past hospitalizations, and medications. We elaborated on the complexity of his limitations, and we made recommendations for an immediate, out of district, therapeutic school placement.

I went into the meeting with my letters tucked away and guns blazing. What struck a chord in me during this meeting was the stark contrast between the cold-hearted classroom teacher and the warmth of the special education team. Honestly, I felt judged by the teacher. I felt her critical gaze assuming that Dave and I didn't know how to discipline our child. The teacher stated she feared for the safety of Joshua's classmates. While I could certainly understand this, I could not understand her unforgiving, icy eyes and lack of compassion. I was unable to find even a tiny glimmer of softness or kindness behind her frozen posture. Her artillery consisted of a notebook documenting Joshua's misbehaviors:

9/12/07

Joshua was out of his chair many times today. He was running around the cabinets and refused to return to his seat. He was very obstinate. The behavior rewards were not working as well today. He was also throwing his crayons when he didn't want to follow the directions, and he was making loud noises. We took him aside many times to talk to him about making better choices. Hopefully he will calm down and get used to his new classroom.

9/13/07

Joshua was very disruptive today. He was also making noises, throwing things, and hitting others. Today he pushed a child at recess and will have to stay in for recess tomorrow. He also went into a teacher's room on the way back from the bathroom. He complains that he is hungry all the time.

9/14/07

This afternoon was difficult for Joshua. After lunch he went to the bathroom accompanied by his aide who stood outside the door. Inside, he hit a boy, then stuffed paper towels in the urinal and then dragged them across the floor. He was also hurting himself with his pencil.

9/15/07

Joshua had a fairly calm morning, but there were still a few flare ups. Today he slammed his desk over. Out of the blue he flipped it over and shoved it across the entire room! We cannot figure out a trigger.

I did not want Joshua with this teacher for another minute. She simply did not have the skills required to deal with Joshua's behavior. After meeting her I became a huge proponent of desensitization training and disability awareness training for regular education teachers interacting with students with special needs. Fortunately, I met Jerry Rigby at this meeting, and he was able to counteract the teacher's cold, impersonal temperament. Jerry had a soft-spoken voice and compassionate eyes, and he spoke to me with concern. Jerry was there to represent his recent creation, the CARE program. This new program was offered from elementary through high school for select students with an emotional disability. It was a therapeutic program designed to meet the emotional, social, and educational needs of these kids.

This placement was a huge blessing because it provided the structure, individualized attention, and emotional support Joshua needed close to home. Mercifully, Joshua would not have to endure long bus rides to an alternative learning program in an unfamiliar city. The team agreed that Joshua was a perfect match for the CARE program. The transition into the program was seamless, and he has been successful in this program ever since.

The CARE program placement had advantages. The classroom never had more than four students and the teacher to student ratio was exceptional! His classroom averaged one teacher, two paraprofessionals, one counselor, and five students. Joshua received the individual and small group attention he needed to flourish. For non-core subjects, Joshua was integrated into a regular classroom with assistance from special education staff.

There were always consistent routines and personalized, behavior management systems, which worked like a charm for Joshua. With accommodations and some creativity, they made learning so much fun! For example, in the winter, science class was outside. Together they all went sledding on the hill behind the school to conduct timed races and learn about nature. Mrs. Shea, the adjustment counselor, was amazing. Joshua felt safe sharing his feelings with her, and she kept in constant communication with me. Mrs. Shea and his teacher Mrs. Thompson found strengths and goodness in Joshua every day, in every way. The most remarkable quality about his teachers and therapists was that they loved Joshua so much. They genuinely *adored* him and embraced him just the way the Lord made him! At the age of eleven, Joshua will be the first student to have completed the program from first through fifth grade—such an accomplishment!

THE EAGLE'S WINGS

Now that Joshua was successfully attending his therapeutic program, behaviors at home temporarily decreased. This luxury provided me with a welcomed opportunity to dig deep down into my heart and focus on my spiritual journey. During this phase, I journeyed into some deep soul searching, most of which was shared with Christi. I journaled a special prayer that I often reflected upon:

> Dear Lord, I was driving into work today and the sun was so brilliant; I yearned to see through the clouds and pretend that piercing brightness was a reflection of heaven. I thought of Moses coming off the mountain with a radiant glow so immense that he needed to cover his face. Today I pray that you will help me have an open, inviting stance in which to receive You. Help me to welcome You regardless of how much or little You provide today.
>
> Please help me have my arms open wide. There are lyrics by David Phelps that sing, "You lived and died….. with arms open wide…" If you can die for me, Jesus, than surely I can have my posture be the same toward you. Amen.

During this period of spiritual inspiration, insight would awaken me at night, and I would also write Christi what was on my heart:

Dear Christi,

Today I sat at church listening to a messaged about "The Timing Test." It correlated closely with the concept of "resting in Him," and I knew I had to share it with you. We live in a world full of instant gratification, Christi. Speed dial, fast food, instant breakfast bars, EZ passes, cell phones, etc! But the Lord has us wait. It seems ironic that we have to wait when He has created man who has come up with ingenious ideas to make things faster and faster. I realized today that I cannot truly wait for things if I am not resting in Him. Psalm 40:1 says, "I waited patiently for the Lord; he turned to me and heard my cry. He lifted me out of the slimy pit, out of the mud and mire; he set my feet on a rock and gave me a firm place to stand."

This is so hard for me to do; my flesh does not want to wait for anything! Not at the Dunkin Donuts line, and certainly not when it comes to waiting for peace to fall upon my son. So many of my prayers for Joshua resonate with the same theme; I pray for peace to fall upon his heart, mind, and soul. Strangely, when I truly wait for the peace I pray for, and I rest in that peace, I am actually at peace without realizing it! Uncanny! Also, by truly resting in God and waiting, I am more prepared for when the Lord does great things in Joshua's and my life—I receive it and appreciate it more.

I realized that the waiting is about his transforming work in my heart and soul. "He who began a good work in you will perfect it until the day of Christ" (Philippians 1:6 (NASB). Pastor Stan said there are three requirements of waiting on the Lord, all of which are not achieved through passive trust. It is only achieved through confident, disciplined, and expectant behaviors. I aspire to have all three of these…do you?

1. (one) Patient trust. Will we be still enough for God's hands to catch us?
2. (two) Confident humility. How often do we remind ourselves we are not in control?
3. (three) Inextinguishable hope. Optimism for what we do not see.

I definitely fall short on these. When my fatigue, doubt, and failures seem too overwhelming, I remind myself of Isaiah 40:28-31:

Do you know? Have you not heard? The Lord is an everlasting God, the Creator of the ends of the earth. He will not grow tired or weary, and his understanding no one can fathom. He gives strength to the weary and increases the power of the weak. Even youths grow tired and weary, and young men stumble and fall. But those who *hope* in the Lord will renew their strength. They will soar on wings like eagles; they will run and not grow weary, they will walk and not be faint.

Wow. Although I have heard this Scripture many times, I find something new to ponder. I struggle with hope as I watch the years go by and yet Joshua continues to suffer. If you also struggle with hope, this scripture holds God's promise to allow you to soar on the wings of an eagle. Have you ever thought of what it means to mount up and soar? There are three ways I can think of.

1. (one) You can flap. Some birds do this frantically—as often as 70-100 times per second.
2. (two) You can glide. Eagles build up speed, then coast for a bit. But with this method you cannot continue for very long.

3. (three) You can soar. Eagles catch columns of air at over 80 mph; it seems they could go forever.

Do you find yourself flapping over and over, constantly working overtime just to stay afloat? Or do you glide by filling your cup full once in a great while, only to peter out quickly because you didn't eat enough worms? Or do you soar? Did Jesus soar on His way to Calvary? Of course not, He could hardly walk with the weight of the cross upon Him! Jesus knows what it is like to struggle and endlessly flap without getting anywhere.

How do we soar like Jesus amidst our pain? It is a simple secret...*hope*. If you cling to hope, Jesus promises you will soar, my friend. Love to you, from your ever flapping, trying to soar, waiting, hoping, allergic, 9/26/72 girlfriend.

THE PERFECT CHRISTMAS TREE

When Joshua was seven-years-old, the Thanksgiving holiday was spent with Dave's parents in Connecticut. After the family feast, the camaraderie came to a close, and we headed back toward Plymouth. With our cocker spaniel Cinamin keeping us company on the car ride, Dave engineered a plan to find our family a Christmas tree at a local evergreen farm. He was very excited to share this experience with the entire family and hoped to create a great memory. Dave found a tree farm in the middle of the country, and thus began our adventure for the ultimate tree cutting experience. A sweet memory was certainly etched in my mind that afternoon!

I tried to withhold my snickering as we began our endeavor; I had this gut feeling things might not go as planned. After all, I knew firsthand what it was like to have my visions of a perfect family experience turn bad. Instead, I quietly tried to support Dave's mission. As we ventured out of our SUV with Cinamin on her leash, the owners of the tree farm offered to let Cinamin run free on their property.

As my eyes scanned the horizon I saw thousands of trees. There were scotch pines, white pines, and douglas firs in perfectly organized rows as far as my eyes could see. The strong scents of Frasier firs wafted through the air, awakening my senses to the delights of the impending holiday season. How to choose? Although it took me only five minutes to find my perfect version of a Christmas tree, I kept quiet because this quick discovery would have made our winter wonderland experience too short. We pressed on, hoping the perfect Bierut tree was waiting for us with a halo of gold wrapped around its top branches.

Our first problem was that since I had been stuck in the car for two hours, I had to go to the bathroom really badly, but we were in the middle of nature. I was distracted from our Christmas tree search because I needed to find a private corner more urgently than the tree. But before I found that perfect spot, we encountered our second problem. I heard Joshua crying across the field; I heard him yelling that his stomach hurt. I looked over his way and saw him crouched on his knees, bent over in the field trying to vomit. I screamed at Joshua to follow me to a more private area. Meanwhile Dave was searching and searching.

Our third problem was that Caleb was obsessed about the hay ride we were *not* there to experience. As the big green tractor slowly passed us by for the third time, Caleb's screams echoed through the fields.

Our fourth problem was that Alexa was in another section of the farm pouting. Developing a strong will and sharp mind of her own, she was convinced that a white spruce was the perfect tree. When Dave told her the needles fall off too quickly, she started giving him the "tude." At this point I had officially checked out and was obsessed with finding an inconspicuous spot to relieve myself.

The fifth problem was Cinamin running like a wild banshee, barking in the fields. Chaos and noise were all around this "peaceful farm."

Finally, Dave screamed, "I wanted this to be perfect! You guys are ruining this for me!" As his voice resonated through the countryside I laughed so hard my stomach hurt. I thought of the fictitious Clark Griswold's family and the pressures we put upon ourselves over the holidays, looking for that perfect family experience. In the end, we were all happy as we made our final decision. We walked off the fields carrying a honking huge, blue spruce. Dave strapped the tree to the top of the SUV, and as we drove into the setting sun, I could see it bouncing resiliently through the sun roof. We survived the drama of the Christmas tree farm.

DOLDRUMS

Holidays are not always what they are cracked up to be. While many people are out shopping, caroling, and spreading good cheer, this December I was struggling again. I felt overwhelmed between my responsibilities at work and as a mother. I just couldn't juggle it all effectively. I felt weary and laden with responsibilities from sunrise to sunset. I felt like I was suffocating; I was exhausted and did not have the energy required to juggle my many roles, relationships, and responsibilities.

During the holidays that year my mom and I watched Alexa perform in the Philharmonic Christmas Concert. My sweet girl had the voice on of angel. While I watched her sing to the gorgeous music, I prayed that the "Christmas spirit" would fill me. But it never came and I did not feel the joy. *Where is it, God?* I thought. For the entire night I found myself inexplicably holding back the tears.

Lord, life is unmanageable right now. Please give me the clarity to change the things I can, and accept the things I cannot change. I don't understand why I feel so blue when I have so many blessings in my life. I prayed.

In the midst of my depression I had a dream where I visited Christi, but her family lived in a different house, and her mom and sister were present for a huge celebration. I wandered and wandered through her beautifully decorated house filled with laughter. I wanted what she had. I longed for the life she had made for herself in Warsaw, Indiana. Abruptly then I awoke, left with only a fuzzy memory of how good it felt to be in her home.

When I shared this little dream with Christi she responded with love and insight. "Jamie, you are in and out of the waters. When you lived her in Warsaw, not unlike your dream, you had the life similar to the life I live now. In your dream, you weren't pining after my life. You were pining after yours."

NONVERBAL LEARNING DISABILITY

Every three years the school district is required to complete a reevaluation for children with special needs to determine their continued eligibility. The school psychologist concluded that at eight years of age, Joshua had a nonverbal learning disability (NVLD), which contributed to his learning and social delays. Although Joshua's intelligence was average, he had a visual-perceptual and visual-motor learning disability as well as problems with communication and social skills.

My years in the school district had already educated me on some of the characteristics that encompass nonverbal learning disabilities. These youngsters may have difficulty interacting with other children and acquiring self-help skills. They are not physically adept, and they are not adaptable. These children bump along (figuratively and literally) through their early elementary years, handling the academic demands fairly well except when their fine motor difficulties get in the way, or they fail to understand the building blocks of addition or subtraction. Many learn better through hearing, rather than seeing (visual processing).

Some children may have difficulty following directions; struggle with math, reading textbooks, and writing essays; continually misunderstand both their teachers and their peers; and become anxious in public and angry at home. They are accused of being lazy, rude, and uncooperative, but nothing could be further from the truth. These children are hardworking, persistent, goal-oriented, and incredibly honest.

Other traits may include the following: great vocabulary, excellent memory, poor organizational skills, trouble with reading comprehension, poor abstract reasoning, weak imaginary skills, physical awkwardness, poor nonverbal communication (gestures, body language), poor social skills, messy handwriting, low self esteem, and trouble adjusting to change (Regents of the University of Michigan, 2011).

I wondered what the difference was between Asperger's disorder and a nonverbal learning disability since Joshua had been diagnosed with Asperger's the prior year. I came to my own humble conclusions regarding this.

- First, a child cannot carry both diagnoses; it's one or the other.
- Second, quite often children are misdiagnosed between the two disabilities.
- Third, both may have an average to above average intelligence.
- Fourth, there are differences with socialization. Many children with Asperger's are happy to be absorbed in their own world; they are content without peer interaction. However, children with NVLD crave that intimacy in relationships, but they do not have the tools to achieve it.
- Fifth, sometimes children with Asperger's are unable to demonstrate empathy, whereas children with NVLD develop empathy more easily.
- Sixth, often children with Asperger's have global developmental delays, while those with NVLD have a specific learning disability that attributes to academic or social delays.

The characteristics associated with NVLD succinctly described Joshua. Joshua definitely possessed empathy, but most of his limitations were invisible. Joshua's inconsistent skill acquisition became incredibly frustrating. Dave yearned for his son to be successful and have the same advantages and skills that he had growing up. Dave could not grasp why Joshua could tie his shoes on Monday but not do it on Tuesday. It didn't make sense that Joshua could utilize eye-hand coordination to eat spaghetti on Wednesday but when leftovers came on Saturday, he literally could not get the food on his fork. No two days were the same; on Monday his fine motor coordination was weak, while on Saturday his hand-eye coordination was weak. Other days it could be his visual-spatial motor skills that prevented his success with making the bed.

Simple activities of daily living such as getting dressed and eating a meal were monumental challenges for Joshua. I resorted to using the software Boardmaker to give him a visual cheat sheet in his bedroom and at the dinner table. The dinner table guide broke down tasks into simple step-by-step directions. I was willing to try anything to have Joshua feed himself successfully and to bring peace for our family mealtime.

This inconsistency drove Dave nearly bonkers. He felt so helpless and frustrated watching Joshua struggle. He believed that the only way to make a difference was to push him to the next level. His heart was in the right place, but his tactics weren't working. Dave's persistence and intensity broke Joshua's spirit to the point where he felt he could never please his father. Dave went through some soul searching during this time and realized that he still struggled with acceptance of Joshua's disabilities. He yearned for his son to live a normal life like any other child.

FEBRUARY BREAK

For the 2009 winter break the entire family drove out to Ohio to stay with my mother. While we were there, I fulfilled my daughterly duties by taking the children to visit their Grandpa Jim for a few hours one morning. After a nice visit with Grandpa Jim, I started preparing Joshua for our departure with ten and five minute warnings. Despite the countdown and negotiations that ensued, Joshua's belligerence left me no choice but to drag him to the car kicking and screaming. I attempted to secure him in his booster seat in the third row of our minivan.

As I drove down the avenue, Joshua unstrapped himself and took off his shoes. He proceeded to climb over the seats and whipped his shoes violently at the back of my head while I was driving. I was beside myself listening to his tirade, and I was fearful for my safety because there was nowhere I could easily pull over the van. When I returned to my mother's house, I ran to Dave and broke into tears while I confided in Dave what had transpired. I feared Joshua thought a new precedent was set for car ride behavior. But he was terribly mistaken.

Later that same day, Dave went along with us to run more errands. On the ride back home, Joshua started raging in the back seat. Again, he managed to unbuckle his seatbelt as he hurled objects toward us in the front. Joshua kicked the seats and screamed wildly. By the time we pulled into my mother's garage, Dave had reached his tipping point. With a voice as deep and loud as the ocean is wide, Dave's yelling reverberated and boomed through the entire home.

I am ashamed to admit that Dave and I are both yellers. We truly have tried everything else, but nothing seemed to grab his attention except a raised voice. We yelled out of desperation and sheer frustration. We yelled, wishing it would give control to a situation that was completely out of our control. And when Dave yelled, his voice was a thousand times scarier and louder than mine.

I don't remember exactly what Dave said to Joshua that day, but I clearly remember Joshua cowering against the rear wheel of the car while my mother watched. She was stunned into silence and frozen in place. She had never seen this side of Dave, and she was catching a magnificent glimpse of our fractured family. I was devastated that I could not control Joshua's behavior and that it took my husband popping a gasket to get Joshua's attention. My mother was disturbed by this scene for weeks.

That week when I visited Christi I tried to put on the façade of the lighthearted best friend. My masquerade did not work; she saw right through me.

"I can see the tiredness behind your eyes, Jamie. Not just physical, but some form of deep-set spiritual weariness. Not depression, but a weariness of heart and soul. Like you've been up all night watching and waiting for morning yet morning isn't coming."

"How can you see into my soul what I am unable to see?" I questioned.

"Jamie, you have an unusual life. Not that I ever thought "normal" was to be strived after, but with Joshy and family and work—and one of those factors would be enough to put "normal" souls over the edge—you have an amazing ability to handle and balance and push forward. At work, you are not just taking on your own emotional issues, but you are reaching out to help other families and take on their pain too. This is a gift you carry, be careful to not let it be a burden."

"But how can I be free of this weariness?" I pleaded.

"Continually give up your concerns and hand them over to God. That is something I am also to do for you. When I pray for you, I am praying in God's will. I just feel so strongly that God is using you to bless others and to further his kingdom and to give God glory. Remember, Joshy is bringing glory to God's name and you are Joshy's mother. "

Christi's wisdom and spot-on assessment of my heart was always accurate, always priceless.

FRANCISCAN'S AT LAST

During late February 2009, Joshua's moods were becoming increasingly difficult to handle, and I found myself at that point where unless I surrendered my own will, I could not manage Joshua's needs and still care adequately for Alexa and Caleb. It was no longer reasonable to sink the entire ship when I couldn't save the one drowning. Joshua took many medications that winter, including lithium, seroquel, Abilify, and strattera. Despite this heavy drug cocktail, his mood was becoming increasingly agitated.

Even more disturbing, I noticed an increase in facial movements and tics. I surmised that these were most likely caused by high doses of seroquel. I was horrified to see the tics because it reminded me of a mild version of the tardiv dyskinesia symptoms again. This concern, paired with the knowledge that some of his medications were at maximum doses, left me resigned that Joshua needed to return to a psychiatric hospital to safely adjust and monitor his medications.

There was no earth shattering crisis or fanfare before this hospitalization. I had learned how to describe Joshua's behaviors as unsafe in effort to secure him a bed somewhere. This time my eye was on the prize—Franciscan Hospital for Children. I was determined to have his psychiatric care at this prestigious facility in Brighton, and I would have waited with him on a gurney in the emergency room for days in effort to make that happen. Thankfully, Franciscan had a bed available and we drove up within hours. We were getting used to the security checkpoints and the pat downs. Joshua could not even wear sneakers with shoelaces due to safety concerns.

There were no pens, no gum, and certainly no jackets with drawstrings allowed.

Every few days I made the trek up to the hospital to spend precious time together. I knew this was an excellent facility, but I would get so riled up each visit when I realized Joshua had other needs that weren't being met. I noticed that the nurses weren't taking care of Joshua's non-psychiatric needs as well. Every time Joshua would greet me he was covered in food on his face and clothing. I worried they were not administering his Flonase for allergies, Miralax for digestion, or Eucerin cream for his eczema.

I hovered over the nurses and teachers. "Did Joshua get his cream today? How many math worksheets did you give him?" Some days the answers were, "No cream, no worksheets." I was incensed. I brought in piles of work from the school and insisted that the special education teacher push through it in effort to prevent more academic delays or, god forbid, having to repeat the school year. It was gut wrenching to see him slide behind when I knew how truly strenuous the work had been for him just to get where he was in school. I could not accept that his entire world beyond this hospital meant *nothing* if we could not control his mood.

When we left him at Franciscan Hospital, I assumed he would stay for a week and then return home to resume life as we knew it. Little did I know Joshua would not return home for almost one month. He entered the hospital moderately sedated due to extremely high levels of seroquel. During this hospitalization, the doctor's first priority was to decrease his sedation and by reducing medications. They weaned him off of the straterra and abilify.

While these were being decreased, they started to titrate up a new medication, Depakote. As the Depakote continued to increase, Joshua started to show more oppositional behavior on the unit. However, the staff was not certain whether his opposition was due to frustration with being away from home, his baseline personality, or more alertness now that he was off of the other drugs. Toward the end of this stay Joshua began wetting the bed again. It was devastating because this became another milestone he worked so hard to accomplish, only to regress again. We were devastated that he had to regress in this area.

CONCUSSIONS

The hospital conducted another EEG and MRI of the brain to look for suspected seizure activity or brain damage, and I was seriously beginning to wonder if they might find something. I remembered the time when Joshua was five and we lived in Pennsylvania. It was during his days of rapid cycling and this particular afternoon he was manic. Joshua and Alexa were playing dress-up in the basement and Joshua chose the superhero costume. He was so caught up in playing pretend, that he started to believe he could fly. Joshua launched himself from the highest basement stair and landed head first onto the concrete floor. He later described, "I went to sleep."

Another concussion happened the previous year at Jellystone Park Campground in Wareham, MA. We were celebrating Alexa's birthday and Joshua had just learned to ride his bike. Praise the Lord he wore a helmet. Apparently Joshua hadn't mastered the craft of slowing down and stopping the bike, so when he went flying down a dirt road with a sharp corner, he crashed head first into a gigantic sycamore tree. Thank God Joshua had the helmet on, but the tree won the battle. As Joshua walked toward me, I thought he was playing a joke on me because the entire left side of his face was hot pink and red. Closer examination left me in a panic as I realized I was looking at mottled chunks of skin. The tree ate the flesh off that side of his face. Within hours the swelling created a baseball-sized lump over his cheek and jaw bone.

I took him home from the party that night, and he started vomiting in my car. His eyes were also dilated, so I rushed him into the emergency room. Miraculously nothing was broken. Yet it was definitely a concussion, and there is still a subtle scar to this day. Needless to say, I was surprised when these new tests all came back negative.

A PROLONGED STAY

S pending two months in a psychiatric hospital is excruciatingly long. They tried to prematurely discharge Joshua after one month, but he lasted back at home for only five days. Each day Joshua's agitation and despair worsened. We quickly contacted Dr. Stromberg and inquired as to whether Josh could return to the hospital. Dr. Stromberg proved to be another one of Joshua's angels. He pulled some strings which allowed Joshua to be remitted immediately without the day-long hassle of going to the emergency room first.

We opted to not tell Joshua he was being readmitted for fear of dangerous behavior while riding in the car. On the long drive up to the hospital, I nervously imagined the moment when Josh would realize he was coming back. I chewed my fingernails to the quick. When we arrived, we were immediately taken back to the conference room with Dr. Stromberg and the case manager. Upon our arrival Joshua admitted feeling very distressed, but otherwise, he was silent. We agreed that the depakote needed to be discontinued, as it appeared to be increasing his agitation. My heart longed to find the perfect medication for him that would work indefinitely. My prayer was that he would never have to be a guinea pig again. We left the intake meeting reluctantly yet resigned certain that Joshua was in the safest place possible.

Back on the unit that first week, Joshua was really struggling. The staff called me to explain he had increased assaultive behavior, which required four episodes of locked-door seclusion and physical holds. When the staff had exhausted all their least restrictive methods to calm him, they called me and asked permission for a chemical restraint. Crying, I gave them permission, for I knew if this qualified staff could not contain him, nobody could. With my consent, the staff administered a shot of thorazine. I was scared of thorazine. Thorazine was used to diminish delusions and hallucinations in schizophrenic patients. This was powerful stuff. If I were to take thorazine, I would be stoned out of this world. They could have set me in a corner for hours drooling all over myself. But for Joshua, who was fueled by adrenaline, it barely scratched the surface of his agitation.

Hours later he finally settled down. He could not even remember why he was upset in the first place. I was so worried about him! I knew the thorazine was meant to help, but I hated myself for agreeing to give it to him. How much could a little body take? Was I poisoning him? *Lord, please send your angels to protect Joshua, him,* I prayed.

After a few weeks went by, we started taking Joshua out for two hour passes. This was an opportunity as a family to spend time together and monitor his behavior. We gauged Joshua's interactions with Alexa and Caleb, his level of compliance, and his ability to go out to a public restaurant or store without becoming over stimulated. During our outings I would bring hair and finger nail clippers to keep him clean. It was the least I could do.

Meanwhile, Joshua was slowly weaned from his depakote, and it was time to start from scratch from a psychopharmacological perspective. The doctor's recommendations were to increase the seroquel to 700 mg and start lamictal. Lamicatal is an anticonvulsant typically prescribed for epilepsy and maintenance treatment for bipolar disorder. Lamicatal must be started slowly and gradually in effort to prevent a potentially lethal rash. We also agreed to restart a new trial of tenex to help with his tics, inattention, and impulsivity.

Through Joshua's prolonged stay at Franciscan, we encountered another predicament. The year prior we purchased a Disney World vacation with nonrefundable airline tickets. As spring break approached, we had to accept that Joshua could not be released from the hospital for the trip. We were torn inside on what to do. How could we leave one child behind? Yet how could we disappoint the other two children and lose thousands of dollars?

After much prayer and counseling from my mother, we decided that we were going to vacation in Disney World without Joshua because she offered to provide an all expenses paid trip to Disney World that fall with just Joshua, me, and her! This was too perfect to pass up. The opportunity to give Joshua individual attention and make his dream come true was staggering. When we broke the news to Joshua that his own trip was being delayed a few months, he took it surprisingly well. Something deep within him knew he needed to remain within the safety of this hospital. We were able to go to Disney World that April knowing that Joshua's grandparents were visiting him, and he was safe within the hospital.

RAINBOW MOON

Christi was always there to inspire me. One time Christi described the night sky as she walked home from her neighbors' house. High above, she witnessed something spectacular—a full moon surrounded by a ring of shadowy clouds with rainbow colors swirling in a perfect circle. She stopped and stared for about ten minutes and then doubted what her eyes were seeing because of its subtlety. But she could not deny its presence; she marveled at its beauty.

Later Christi heard on the news that there had been a rainbow moon for a *brief time* that evening. Rainbow moons are extremely rare. The human eye sees incredible colors and swirls creating a ring around the moon. This phenomenon occurs when light passes through six-sided ice crystals high in the atmosphere. These crystals, dubbed diamond dust, can be quite complex with multiple concentric circles, arcs, and portions of arcs all arrayed in spectacular geometric designs (Kevin Cooley, 2011).

Christi praised God. "I saw it! I was probably one in a million who had seen it!"

She asked God why she was lucky enough to see the moon rainbow.

He answered her, "Because you looked *up*."

This made me wonder how often I looked up to see what God was putting directly in front of me. Christi reminded me that God sees me as He sees Joshua—one in a million. The rainbow moon was something I was always searching for. I've never seen this mysterious phenomenon, and probably will not until I get to heaven. Or have I? Is my rainbow moon in front of me every day? Is my rainbow moon my one in a million children? Is it Joshua? Is it the fascination and awe that washes over me when Joshy lovingly melts into my arms with a good morning hug? Or maybe it's in the love letter for Mother's Day that he diligently worked on for an entire week?

I was reminded of my rainbow moon when I read Joshua's painstaking, childlike handwriting. It served as a reminder of how tremendous his heart was and how desperate he needed to show me he loved me.

> My mom is special because she is talented. She is a good cook. I like to play games with my mom. We like to go to the beach together. I will make her mother's day special by taking her out to dinner. Happy Mother's Day, Mom!
>
> Love, Josh

First Signs of Lyme

With new insight about my own rainbow moons, I cherished each of my children for being that one in a million. I promised the Lord to look up for answers, and I paid closer attention to people and circumstances the Lord put in my path.

I really trusted in Dr. Stromberg and believed the Lord put him in Joshua's life for a reason. Dr. Stromberg wanted to rule out every possible reason for Joshua's agitation. One seemingly random test he ordered was the Western Blot Lyme Disease Titer in effort to rule out Lyme disease.

Initially I doubted Joshua was carrying Lyme antibodies. It seemed like Dr. Stromberg was taking stabs in the dark. However, Newton-Wellesley Hospital Laboratory immediately returned the results with a presumptive positive for Lyme antibodies. The report indicated Joshua had positive IgG antibodies on bands P18, P30, P39, P41, P58, P66, and P93. Their impression: "Consistent with infection with Borrelia burgdorferi at some time in the past" (Newton-Wellesley Hospital, 2009). The results required an automatic second test for Lyme titers by the MAYO medical laboratory.

Two weeks later the MAYO laboratory's serology results returned. Indeed, private records confirmed that while IgM antibodies are produced immediately after exposure to the disease, IgG antibodies are created a few months later. This was how the toxicologists knew the infection was not recent. Confirmation of Joshua's Lyme disease was mandated reportable to the Center for Disease Control (CDC). The enormity of this discovery was slowly sinking in. Dr. Stromberg was not a specialist in this area, so he contacted infectious disease consultants. They recommended Joshua be taken to New England Medical Center (NEMC) for further evaluation surrounding the possibility of central nervous system involvement. They were attempting to discover if the Lyme disease had caused an active infection, manifested as encephalitis or meningitis.

An MRI of the brain and a lumbar puncture (spinal tap) was required. The logistics of getting this accomplished were complicated and taxing. We had to leave Plymouth at five in the morning and temporarily discharge Joshua from Franciscan in order to take him to NEMC for the day for testing. We ventured through Boston rush hour traffic and arrived at NEMC by eight. Once we settled in, Joshua was prepped for sedation and carted away for testing. The procedures lasted a few hours, but it took many more for Joshua to awaken. Exhausted, we returned him to the unit at Franciscan late that evening. Now it was a waiting game.

The next week the results came back negative for an active infection in the brain or blood. I knew this was wonderful news, but I couldn't help but wonder, "What's next?" I asked the physicians at NEMC about treatment options. They explained that since Joshua's exposure to Lyme was not recent and an active infection was not in his central nervous system, there was *no* course of recommended action. This did *not* set well with me. At that time I did not know much about Lyme disease, but I had heard if it was not treated, one can experience a lifetime of joint pain. I had also heard that antibiotics are a recommended course of action against the bacteria.

I confronted the medical team about my concerns for Joshua's long term health. The doctors replied, "Well, we thought you might ask about that. If you want, we can write a prescription for three weeks of antibiotics."

"Is that going to help him get better?"

"We doubt it. If Lyme disease is not caught immediately, we do not believe there is any effective treatment that exists. But we'll prescribe some antibiotics it if you would like." Angrily, I retorted, "I do not want you to prescribe him something just to *humor* me! I want you to offer him treatment to make him better! Forget your stupid antibiotics!"

I just loved hearing yet another diagnosis with no options for treatment. This couldn't be possible. There has to be somebody or something out there that can allow my son a more promising future.

While I waited for the results from the lab I started putting the puzzle pieces together. It was complicated connecting a timeline to Joshua's medical and psychiatric symptoms. When did Joshua get Lyme disease? I knew he had to have been bitten by an infected deer tick a long time ago. But *when?* It all started rushing back; images flooded my mind. Joshua certainly was a happy baby that first year of life, but then something changed when he turned one. I certainly remembered camping with Joshua when he was a baby, but I couldn't fathom that Lyme disease was prevalent in the golden wheat fields of Indiana back then. I gradually accepted that it took only one forest, one contaminated deer tick, and one host- my darling little baby rolling through the grasses—to contract this disease.

Joshua was hospitalized or taken to specialists with those mystery illnesses at ages two, four, and six, all with no explanation for the cause of his rashes and joint pain. They tested him for Lyme back in Pennsylvania, but he had just finished a full course of antibiotics for an upper respiratory infection. Even if he didn't get the disease in Indiana, we did move to Pennsylvania on the outskirts of the Poconos Mountains. Hmm…He never had that bulls-eye rash the professionals often refer to. Could this disease be the cause of his symptoms? Really, truly?

INSIDIOUS

The first thing I discovered was that there were twenty-six cases of Lyme disease reported in Indiana during 2001, and there has been a steady increase every year since (Centers for Disease, 2011). The CDC also claims that 60 percent of untreated Lyme cases will result in arthritis later in life (Allen C. Steere, 2001).

Lyme disease (LYD) is a multisystem illness caused by the tick-borne spirochete Borrelia burgdorferi (Bb). The CDC requires that five bands are present to warrant a diagnosis of Lyme exposure; IGenX Labratories only requires two bands to be present. Joshua had seven; he blew both criterions out of the water. Sadly, there are many people who do not meet the CDC criteria yet have many debilitating symptoms of Lyme disease. These cases go unreported, as do many undetected cases, resulting in a much higher prevalence than the CDC's reports.

For those who recognize immediate infection by discovery of the tick attached to the body or a bulls-eye rash, a three week supply of antibiotics usually eradicates the disease. However, there are many who go undiagnosed or misdiagnosed, and "...children are the most vulnerable to its effects. Often going misdiagnosed in the early stages, children can suffer complications from Lyme and tick-borne diseases like seizures, crippling arthritis, and developmental disorders. With proper treatment, though, even the most severely afflicted can go on to live healthier lives." When exposure is left untreated for months or years, chronic Lyme disease can develop (*http://www.lymesite. com/Dr%20Jones%20why%20give%20support.htm*).

EPIPHANY

As I continued my research on the impact of chronic Lyme disease, something striking stood out to me: *Every single symptom Joshua has presented with his entire life has been documented as a possible characteristic of chronic Lyme disease.* All the "alphabet soup" jargon Joshua was labeled with actually fit in a neat and tidy package under this umbrella.

I still believed that Joshua presented with many clinical manifestations of other disorders (i.e. NVLD, ADHD), but did he *really* have those disabilities, or were they a byproduct of a disease caused by a resilient, infected, microscopic deer tick?

There are multiple cognitive problems associated with the disease, all of which have a significant impact on learning and school performance. This includes difficulty with attention and concentration; speed and efficiency of processing information; learning and memory; auditory processing and language expression, planning and organization, and multitasking.

Other manifestations of Lyme disease described Joshua perfectly. His symptoms and abilities were always waxing and waning, always unpredictable from day to day. His mood instability, exhaustion, and trouble with expressing his thoughts could all be attributed to the disease. The inexplicable joint pain and rashes, poor memory, confusion, and attention deficits were also documented.

I was stunned that we finally found the missing puzzle piece after all these years. And as usual, Christi was there to help me process the new information about my precious son. She reminded me how to extract the precious from the worthless. Christi convinced me that God's grace extends to all of us despite our strengths or weaknesses. She helped me see that the word "disabled" is not in God's vocabulary when he speaks or thinks or loves His children. Instead, God is in the business of extracting the precious from the worthless. God wanted to restore in me His perspective of Joshy's "precious" no matter the disability. I was finally at a place where I could understand that God reveals Himself uniquely and there is a special place for these children who are weak.

OUR ANGEL

I was quickly realizing that there was a lot of research on Lyme disease that needed to be done, and I desperately needed to find somebody who was willing to help my son. God, with his sovereignty, showed me exactly where to go at just the right time. That week New England's television station Chronicle was interviewing Dr. Charles Ray Jones, a pediatric Lyme specialist, from New Haven, Connecticut, only three hours away from where we lived.

Dr. Jones' website quotes the following: "For years, Dr. Jones has put everything on the line to help children regain their health. Now in his eighties, he still dedicates his life to protecting the most vulnerable among us. One of a small handful of physicians in his line of work, he puts in an incredible number of hours each week with the mission of preventing the suffering of sick children" (http://www.drjoneskids.org, 8/10/11).

I confided to my girlfriend, Karen, about my suspicions that Joshua contracted Lyme disease when he was a mere baby and how there was supposedly this "miracle worker" in Connecticut. Karen admitted she felt the Holy Spirit prodding her to encourage me down this path. She was emphatic about our opportunity to meet Dr. Jones. Karen confirmed my growing belief that Lyme disease could be the impetus behind what made Joshua tick (no pun intended!). I was determined not to ignore what God was placing before me. I was looking for my rainbow moon. I found Dr. Jones' number on the internet and easily made the initial appointment, but I was disappointed that it was going to take nearly six months to get in! They explained to me that the wait was long because families from *all over the world* fly in to see Dr.

Jones. I was filled with hope and anticipation when I thought of meeting this doctor. I explained Joshua's complicated history to the nurse on the telephone, and filled with compassion, she gave me an appointment from the cancellation list. Surprisingly, we received a call the very next week! Joshua's first visit was on a cool, crisp, October day. Adrenaline pumping, I ventured out on the three hour journey toward New Haven, soon to become a memorized travel route. I geared up for the trip with drinks, snacks, and Joshua's Nintendo DS.

When we finally arrived at Dr. Jones' office, we were introduced to perhaps the warmest, gentlest, elderly man in this world, let alone amongst the profession of doctors. At first I was concerned that he appeared so haggard and old. I was not used to physicians sitting behind their desk in sweatpants. As he hobbled over to greet me, I guessed his age to be mid eighties.

Although Dr. Jones could not hear well, he quickly proved he was smart as a whip with his razor sharp mind. Perhaps the best part of this encounter was that Joshua was completely smitten, head over heels enamored with Dr. Jones. Children tend to have internal radar that helps them discern who is or is not safe, and Joshua absolutely melted that day; he instinctively knew Dr. Jones would never hurt him.

After a thorough exam and lengthy discussion, we decided to begin treatment with baseline antibiotics. Dr. Jones described that the deadly spirochetes created had infested Joshua's entire body; they had burrowed themselves throughout his blood, his organs, and his brain. These crafty boogers had even protected themselves in these areas by putting up individualized armored walls around themselves. The spirochetes didn't want to leave the comfort of its host. They were like parasites, sucking away the high quality functioning of his body and brain.

Dr. Jones further explained that long term, antibiotic treatment, though controversial, was the only way to break through the spirochetes' seemingly impenetrable barriers. I imagined the antibiotics to be like the armored vehicles in the movie *Armageddon*. They were swift and adept at thrusting their long penetrating drills deep into the deadly meteor floating in space. They were going to blast it away.

That initial appointment lasted two hours and cost seven hundred dollars that insurance would not cover. Subsequent appointments were $325, but it continues to be worth it. I left the office that day feeling something special I hadn't experienced in years – newfound hope. Who can put a price tag on hope?

When we started Joshua on antibiotics, we noticed changes immediately. The first things to improve were his speech articulation, attention, and mood. A few weeks later, his fine motor skills improved. After another week, his processing speed and ability to perform multi-step directions improved. But most importantly, Joshua was happier. He didn't have to try so darn hard for everything. Learning wasn't as difficult, and regulating his mood was easier. It was spine-tingling and absolutely electrifying to see a miracle like this happen before our eyes!

Ecstatic, I thought about shouting it out to the world! I dreamed aloud to Dave, "Do you think I should contact that show, Mystery Diagnosis? Or I should I get an agent to secure us a spot on The Doctors? And while I'm at it, I may as well try for the 700 Club!

Second Visit

Our next appointment was three months later. About one month before that time, Joshua's rapid improvements started to level out. The morning of our departure, I admit I had a terrible attitude. All I could focus on was the dreadful six hours of traveling required. It really exhausted me. When I dropped Caleb off at church so Pastor Stan could watch him, I saw a friend in the parking lot who offered to pray for me before we left. It was that prayer that turned my day around. Oh the sweet power of prayer! She prayed for travel mercies, my attitude, Joshua's comfort, and for medical miracles to continue.

When we saw Dr. Jones, I explained to him how I had been on an emotional rollercoaster after seeing such incredible gains that eventually tapered off. He put my fears to ease and explained that this was common through the process; it only meant that we were learning more about what medication worked best long term for Joshua.

Dr. Jones shared with me more about his life's mission to help children suffering with this disease. The more I learned, the more amazed I became at the adversity this man has had to overcome. He was truly inspiring. I believed with all my heart that the Lord brought me to Dr. Jones to inspire me and provide hope. Meeting him was the closest experience I'll ever have to meeting somebody on earth like Mother Theresa. At a complete sacrifice to his health, finances, time, and family, Dr. Jones continued his mission to help those less fortunate.

Dr. Jones assured me that he had helped many children like Joshua who had prior diagnoses on the autistic spectrum and existed only within in their own world. One time, a mother brought in her little boy who had an autism diagnosis. This little boy rarely spoke, especially not to strangers. During that visit, Dr. Jones held the boys' chin in the palm of his hands and promised the boy, "I am going to unlock the key to your brain." The boy was given antibiotics.

When the family returned three months later, Dr. Jones welcomed them into his office. The little boy recognized Dr. Jones and gingerly approached him. Next, the boy placed his hands on both sides of Dr. Jones' cheeks, and said, "Thank you for unlocking the key to my brain." As Dr. Jones told me a riveting story with tears in his eyes which which left me in awe. Here was a little boy who never spoke, only to be speaking in sentences three months later! The Lord truly blesses some physicians with extraordinary wisdom and passion to help the meek and mild. Dr. Jones does Jesus proud. When we left this second visit, not only was I filled with hope again, but so was Joshua.

We arrived back in Plymouth late that evening where Dave, the kids, and our friends were at worship practice. I rushed in and asked them to pray with me on Joshua's behalf. Eagerly we held a prayer vigil and placed Joshua in the center of our circle. Together we prayed a vehement prayer for continued healing at the doctor's hands.

It was late when we got home, but we were so full of the Holy Spirit. I instructed the boys to get ready for bed, but Joshua turned to me and said, "Wait!" When I looked at him, for the first time in his life, with tears in his eyes, *he looked me directly in the eye* and said, "Mommy, thank you for everything you've done for me. I love you." In that instant, I knew that every battle we had endured together was worth it. In that moment, I knew that our souls were meant to collide with each other. That spring we enjoyed Joshua's progress in all areas and continued to feel God's grace lavished upon us.

GRANDPA JIM

June 3, 2009 was a day I will never forget. It was my cherished firstborn's birthday! This year Alexa was turning eleven-years-old, approaching the cusp of those magical teenage years. I couldn't have been more proud of the young woman she was becoming. My mother and sister were visiting that week in anticipation of a big celebration. Before the fun could begin that evening, I needed to put in a few hours of work over at the school that morning. I had planned to escape work right after lunch so I could decorate the house and pick up her cake.

As I was finishing up at the special education department's administrative offices, my phone rang. When I saw Dad appear on the screen I thought, Darn him! He never calls, and when he does it's in the middle of my workday! Despite the inconvenience, I longed to hear his scratchy, baritone voice.

"Hi Dad, I'm at work. What's up?"

He only replied with "Hi, honey," and then dead silence.

"Dad, is everything okay? Why aren't you talking?"

"Well, honey, actually everything is *not* okay." Another long pause ensued until he uttered, "Jamiekins, this is the most difficult phone call I've ever made in my entire life. Honey, remember the pain that I mentioned a few weeks ago? It was pain in my abdomen which wrapped around my side. You told me to get checked out, remember? Well, I didn't tell you I was also having trouble eating and swallowing. Last week I finally went to the doctor and I've been having tests done."

Quickly grasping where this conversation was headed, I interjected, "What is it dad? Tell me!" His voice was heavy with reservation and weariness.

"Honey, I have cancer."

"No, you don't!" I spit out, "Are you serious?"

"You know I would never joke about something like this. I have stage four esophageal cancer, and it has spread to my liver. The doctor said I don't have much time, honey. It looks like this is going to be a short trip."

I started sobbing in front of my colleague; I felt my head swirl and the room spin.

"What are your options, Dad?"

"Well, there are options such as chemotherapy or surgery, but my cancer is too advanced; it may only prolong my life by a few months. The doc says I have two to six months at most. Jamie, please go home and tell your sister and mother, then call me so I can talk to all three of you together. I love you to pieces."

As I hung up the phone, I was flooded with emotion. My adrenaline was surging as I began ranting and raving to God. The voices inside of my head screamed, *Lord, how can You do this to me? My father is only sixty-two. He's too young to die! My children need their Grandpa Jim and I still need my daddy!*

During my drive home from work, I made a feeble attempt at pulling myself together. First I called Dave for emotional support. Next, I called home and asked my mother and sister to meet me outside *without* the kids. I was trying to protect the children from the drama that would unfold. As I pulled in the driveway, I could see their guarded looks full of curiosity. I walked to over to them under our basketball hoop. In that moment that hoop only reminded me of the special time I shared with my father playing basketball when I was a little girl.

With a big gulp, I spilled the news, "Dad has terminal cancer. He only has a few months to live." Shocked, we stood there crying as we huddled in our small circle. We leaned on each other's shoulders and stood united as a family once again, knowing my father was going to need us all. The day was pretty much ruined by this tragic news, but we managed to keep our chins up for Alexa's sake. Secretly, I feared that on every future birthday, I would always associate it with being the beginning of the end for my father rather than the blessing of Alexa's life.

We all agreed Jessica and Mom should return immediately to Ohio so they could be with my father. Despite an incredibly bitter divorce between my parents in 2000, my mom's renewed faith and time healed many wounds. Both managed to find forgiveness and remain friends. They spent over thirty years together, so a piece of each of their hearts would always love each other.

I crumbled to pieces as Mom and Jessica drove away. I called Christi while I lay beside the barberry bushes on the side lawn. I wept as I shared my tragic news with her. We remembered a time many years prior when Christi, Mary, and I had a powerful prayer session on behalf of my father. That night Christi was struck with a sense of urgency for my father's health and salvation. During our prayers, the Lord revealed to Christi that my father's time was short.

I never asked her back then just how short, but as I sat on the lawn gasping for air. Sniffling, I asked Christi, "What sort of a time frame did God put upon your heart that night many years ago?"

Quietly she responded, "About eight years."

Together we counted back the years since our prayer vigil in Indiana—eight years exactly.

From the moment my mom and sister left, I felt desperate and alone. I struggled with living so far away from my family; I felt lost without them. *Why do I always have to be the one living so far away?* I cried. As much as I loved Plymouth, my heart was breaking at the thought of being unable to help out my family and be with dad in his final days. When mom's second husband, John, died of lung cancer, I wasn't there. When my grandmother and grandfather died, I wasn't there. *I wasn't there.* There just had to be a way.

LEAVING MY BABIES

The next day Pastor Stan called me to express his prayers and provide encouragement. I shared how torn I was because I knew my family needed me in Plymouth, but God laid it upon my heart to spend my summer with my father caring for him in his final days. Pastor Stan proposed a magnificent solution for my dilemma. He suggested that I consider hiring his twenty-year-old son, David, as our nanny for the summer. The timing was completely orchestrated by God. David was scheduled to arrive home from college the next day, and did not need to return until September.

I stood amazed at how the pieces fell into place. Not only was David a wonderful, energetic, godly man, but he was simply amazing with Joshua! I could not imagine anyone better equipped to leave with my kids. David was able to take Joshua to psychiatry appointments, the Camp Clark bus, beaches, ponds, and stores. When my mother offered to pay for David's services, the deal was sealed. God removed every obstacle and opened every door to enable me to be with my father.

I quit my job without a second thought. Now I had *two* people to care for, one being half way across the country. I left the next day. I felt such a mixture of emotion—gratitude, trepidation, and heartsickness. I was grateful for Dave because he supported my decision to be with my father, which meant he had to work full time and raise the children alone. There was trepidation as well because Dave and I had never been apart for more than one week over the past twelve years. I was weary of being separated for that long. I was also heartsick to leave my three babies behind. I knew children were resilient, but they just had no concept of how long I would be gone, and Joshua's unpredictability made me nervous. I had to leave it all in God's hands.

TICS

That first week I was in Ohio, Dave mentioned to me that Joshua's tics were getting much worse. Without seeing it myself, I simply told him to keep an eye on it. But one week later Dave drove out the children to stay with me while he went on a business trip. The elation of hugging my babies was snuffed out as I watched the scene before me. There was my beautiful boy, ecstatic to see me, but unable to hug me. Joshua was erratically jerking and twitching all over the place. He was also constantly clearing his throat, blinking his eyes, and jerking his head sideways. His torso even convulsed and twitched in rhythmic waves so it looked like he was doing the worm dance. Most alarming, his breathing was pressured and inconsistent. He could not complete a simple task like eating or sleeping.

It appeared that tardiv dyskinesia had returned with a vengeance due to the extremely high Seroquel dosage Joshua was taking. The gravity of his medical situation began to sink in; we were half way across the country, from our team of experts. Desperately I prayed for God to take control of what was clearly beyond my limited resources. Next, I paged Mary Ann and typed in 911. She returned my call immediately and informed me that Joshua had a tough road ahead of him. Due to the severity and potential permanence of the tardiv dyskinesia symptoms, we had to purge his body of Seroquel right away. "Throw it down the toilet" she instructed. Quickly I witnessed the dire consequences which occur when somebody abruptly stops taking high dosages of Seroquel.

Mary Ann prescribed Cogentin and Ativan to combat the tremors. The first night I gave Joshua the Ativan in attempt to stop his arms from flailing so he could fall asleep. Since the prescription stated he could have two doses if one was not effective, after Joshua was still suffering thirty minutes later I gave him the second dose. My mother's and my hearts were absolutely broken; we wanted to take away his pain.

Joshua just couldn't drift off to sleep. Finally he emerged from his bedroom at ten that evening. Crying, he claimed there were scary things flying in the air. Joshua saw The Cat in the Hat, a litter of kittens, and random objects floating around. Joshua had an adverse reaction from the Ativan which was causing hallucinations. I swept him into my arms and carried him off to my bedroom; we were going to have to brace this storm together. Never leaving his side, I stayed up with Joshua as he thrashed and hallucinated all night. By four in the morning, merciful sleep finally fell upon his tortured body and mind.

Another medication meant to help Joshua only hurt him. I grieved for him and wished for him a normal, healthy childhood. I prayed for the pain to become my own. Joshua awoke after ten that morning, and I mistakenly thought the worst was behind us. Quickly Joshua ran into the bathroom to vomit. This continued every thirty minutes throughout the day. With all five senses on high alert, I experienced electrifying sizzles up and down my spine while I grasped the severity of this Seroquel withdrawal. I prayed, "Sweet Jesus, this just isn't fair! Please, I beg of You, comfort my son! Take me instead Lord! Give me his pain!" Twenty-four hours later, the worst had subsided, but my mother, Joshua, and I were physically and emotionally exhausted. Most importantly, the tics had greatly diminished and he was breathing better. Even still, I resented that this travesty had to happen the one and only week Joshua was in Ohio to say goodbye to his dying grandfather. Yet my heart also knew that the Lord brought him to me so I could help him through the inevitable suffering he was to endure.

GOODBYES

By the time Dave returned to Ohio, he could not tell the living hell Joshua experienced. Reluctantly Dave and I took the children to say their final goodbyes to Grandpa Jim. Crocodile tears flowed, but mercifully it seemed that Joshua understood that death was really a new beginning in heaven. Gently I explained to Joshua that Grandpa Jim had accepted Jesus in his heart and would be waiting for us someday when it was our turn. I wondered if Joshua's young mind grasped the reality that he was never going to see him again. Yet my subsequent goodbye with Joshua was more painful, evidenced by profuse crying and screaming. He missed me terribly.

To shorten my total time away from home, I returned to Massachusetts for a visit in late July for Joshua's ninth birthday. I had Dave arrange for us to stay in a hotel in Boston before we returned to Plymouth so that we could reconnect. I could not wait to see my man! At the airport I literally jumped into his arms and wrapped my legs around him, just like in the movies. But after working full time and filling my shoes the past month, poor Dave was exhausted. We ate dinner at a nice restaurant and then he fell asleep in five minutes, no joke. He slept like a baby. I think he deserved that.

My father died on August 25, 2009. That day heaven's gates opened up to greet their newest angel into their celestial realm. His emotional and physical suffering on earth ended. Revelation 21:4 promises, "The Lord will wipe every tear from their eyes. There will be no more death or mourning or crying or pain, for the old order of things has passed away." Another special man disappeared and drifted out of Joshua's life.

FINAL HOSPITALIZATION

The summer before Joshua entered the fourth grade I opted Joshua out of attending summer school. For the past three years, Joshua had gone to summer school, yet he still regressed by every fall. Although the consistency summer school provided was beneficial, it also meant missing beach trips, pool days at Grammy's, Vacation Bible School, and Camp Clark. I believed these experiences were equally important for his development. I admit I also felt a twinge of guilt because I missed the entire summer with my children the year prior while taking care of my father. This was my first venture with home schooling so I plunged right in. And then I wobbled right back out!

In that short time, I developed a new respect for all special education teachers and therapists. It was ambitious trying to keep a daily routine for Joshua while his siblings wanted to run to the beach and watch cartoons. It was even more problematic trying to get Joshua to focus while his siblings were playing outside and the dogs were barking! I stunk at teaching my own child; I became frustrated. I couldn't understand why one day Joshua could master a complex math equation, while the next he could not compute a simple problem like $5 + 8 = 13$.

Thankfully I had a behavior management program that was working for the boys. Since Joshua's maturity level was close to Caleb's, I figured I had to treat them like twin six-year-old boys. I devised a stop light system with a behavior chart where they earned rewards for good behavior. My behavior system required constant monitoring, and eventually I grew lazy.

Although I could get the boys to listen to me, I could not stop the fighting. The fighting between the three children was vicious and cruel. A discouraged, melancholy spirit washed over me as I wondered what price God wanted me to pay in order to maintain some peace in my home. I wrongfully coveted peace above my relationship with God. I pined for my own inner peace, hoping that it would trickle down into the kids, but after the twentieth fight in one hour, I would snap. The bitter reality was that I had three beautiful, kind, warm, loving children individually, but together they were toxic. Neither shared similar interests or personalities and they brought out the worst in each other. I pleaded with God that summer Psalm 19: 4 (NLT), "Let the words of my mouth and the meditation of my heart be pleasing to you." I couldn't achieve this alone; I had to rely on Him every step of the way.

I tried to cling to this prayer but it became harder and harder as the fighting escalated. By August Joshua was absolutely beside himself. Out of pure desperation, he started threatening Caleb, "I hate you. I'll kill you!" he screamed. Soon the fists started flying, and I realized Joshua was threatening the safety of others, and he was clearly miserable. When I spoke with Dr. Stromberg at Franciscan Hospital he agreed that a short inpatient stay may be necessary in order to tweak the medications in a safe environment.

In hindsight, I regretted this decision; I blamed myself for not being able to handle the children's fighting better that summer. I still played the "if only" game with my choices. *If only I had more patience, we could have worked this out at home. If only I had a better behavior system in place, Joshua wouldn't have felt desperate. If only I wasn't so selfish with my time, then I would have recognized the warning signs earlier!* The astounding responsibilities paired with my insecurities nearly crippled me. Most children have screamed at one time or another that he hates his brother or wants to kill his sister, but when a child with a history of mood imbalance makes that statement the parent must respond differently.

My heart knew that Joshua would never have acted on those impulsive words, but I used him as our scapegoat. The truth was that our family was in such disequilibrium that getting Joshua the immediate help that was available to him seemed the quickest and simplest route. It was a small consolation that Joshua went back to a familiar hospital, but visiting him never became easier. The joys of the reunion were shattered by the sorrows of goodbye. The first weekend of Joshua's stay, he received a pass that enabled him to do something special off grounds with his family.

We were eager for the day together because we were acting as tourists in Boston. We were taking a Duck Tour of the city then dining at Fire and Ice that evening! Joshua was so content to be back with his family. I wondered how I could surrender him to the hospital again that night. After an amazing day full of laughter and fun, we unenthusiastically embraced goodbye with tears dripping down our cheeks. I knew Joshua would be back at home where he belonged in only a few more days, but it never took away the sting as we drove away.

Despite my best and worst motherly intentions to control Joshua's world, this hospitalization reminded me how difficult it was to decipher when to intervene and when to let go. The tough reality was that I was not his primary caregiver during his stay at Franciscan. There were so many small ways in which I cared for Joshua which I had to release control. *Who will pray with him tonight, Lord? Who will remind him to wipe his mouth after every bite?* I prayed. Slowly I began to accept that everything was in God's hands. Psalm 121 reassured me that the Lord "watches over you…he watches over you….now and forever." *Dear Lord, I'm clinging to this promise. Watch over my child while he's away.* I prayed.

CMT 1A

Joshua was always a toe walker. Not only did he walk on his tippy toes, but for the last few years, he would also clench and curl under his toes. Although I warned Joshua that he could get painfully disfigured hammer toes, he could not stop clenching them. It was an autonomic response that he had no control over. During the summer of 2009, Joshua had a growth spurt and his feet became severely crooked, disfigured, painful, and weak.

Alarmed, I took him to the local podiatrist. She took one look at his feet and refused to treat him until he had a neurological consultation first. I was so annoyed! I had already taken Joshua for this type of assessment before. I didn't understand its significance. I begrudgingly escorted Joshua to another neurologist on the Cape who did nothing more than craft a report on Joshua's life story.

Still, his feet were degenerating quickly. I realized he needed the big guns and I set up an appointment with Dr. Mahan, one of the top pediatric orthopedic foot surgeons, at Boston's Children's Hospital. She was amazing. After five minutes of observation, she shared with me that she suspected the cause of the foot deformities from Charcot-Marie tooth disease otherwise known as CMT 1A. Dr. Manhan immediately sent us down to neurology to have an electromylogram (EMG) test on all four extremities. The test revealed that Joshua's reflexes in both his hands and feet were unresponsive to stimuli, which is an indicative sign of CMT 1A. Genetic testing was submitted quickly thereafter, and within three weeks the results came back positive. Now on top of everything else, Joshua had been diagnosed with a degenerative, neurological disease. I cried out to God in angst and misery on behalf of my son's suffering. But Joshua never complained. Not a single, solitary time.

CMT affects approximately one in twenty-five hundred people in the United States. It is an inherited neurological condition which causes peripheral neuropathy. CMT 1A disrupts the myelin sheath surrounding axons responsible for nerve conduction. Because the conduction is delayed, the nerves cannot transmit their signals then to the muscles and sensory organs in the limbs. With CMT1A, the gene is often duplicated (though there are many other variations) on chromosome seventeen that carries the instructions for producing the peripheral myelin protein-22 (PMP-22). Symptoms include weakness, tingling, numbness, and pain in the hands and feet. Minimal reflexes are present. Foot drop, claw toe, ankle and foot muscle atrophy, high arches, and hammer toes are associated. Symptoms are exacerbated over time, leading to debilitation of the hands and feet if left untreated ("Charcot-Marie-tooth," 2011). Although it was incredulous that Joshua had yet another disability, the diagnosis did encompass his symptoms. Now I understood why, despite *years* of therapy, his fine motor skills, weak grasp, hand and foot pain, decreased coordination, and his clumsiness and tripping were not improving.

Dr. Mahan explained that correcting Joshua's feet was an urgent matter and that surgery was necessary to rebuild the strength and function in Joshua's feet. As humble as Dr. Mahan's demeanor appeared, I knew the truth. She was offering my son a better quality of life. She was after all, one of the hospital's miracle makers. Dr. Mahan promised Joshua's feet would be healed for at least the next twenty years or longer. No more excessive tripping, no more lethargy with running, improved balance and coordination, and much less pain. How could I not pursue this promise for Joshua's future?

As the realization set in that Joshua's feet were truly disfigured and limiting, I feared for his future. *How cruel is it to physically limit a boy with so much energy?* I thought. But late at night, in the middle of sweet slumber, God sent me a spiritual dream that stripped me of my anxieties. It was an odd dream which didn't make any logical sense without investigation into the symbols from the Bible.

The concept was simple: a bear transformed into a lion, and then a deer frolicked on top of this beast while it lay there in complete surrender. In scripture, bears and lions are portrayed as beasts of prey equipped with ferocity and cunning. But when Daniel was thrown into the lions' den he emerged without wounds because he trusted God to save his life. Through this story I realized I did not have to live in fear of the beasts (Joshua's illness) any longer because God would continue to cover and protect Joshua.

The deer set free in my dream reminded me of the expression, "A doe set free bears beautiful fawns." *Was I the doe, destined to be set free?* I questioned. God was gently prodding me to surrender my insecurities for what was out of my control. Upon doing so, He would free me from the bondage of my doubt in His ability to help Joshua. As I thought about Joshua's feet, I remembered Isaiah 35:6 states, "The lame will leap like a deer." I linked this verse to Habakkuk 3:19, "The sovereign Lord is my strength. He makes my feet like the feet of a deer and enables me to go on the heights." Guess what? In my dream, the fawns frolicked with joy.

Joshua—my fawn—will leap like a dear and frolick with joy. Of one thing I am certain: God was telling me to *trust Him* and that *He will heal my son and restore my faith in this matter.*

COMPLEX CARE

ach of Joshua's feet needed two phases of surgery, the first being scheduled for January 2011. In the meantime, I was drowning in the medical system. While I prided myself on being able to navigate the social services network for my child, I was unexpectedly tossed into the world of doctors, therapists, and hospitals at the same time. I found myself at the mercy of muzac on phone lines, disconnected calls, and hours of traveling to and from appointments.

Recently Joshua had gotten some lab results in from Quest Diagnostics which flagged that he had very low immunoglobulin levels. Appointments were made with the immunology team at Children's. They sent us back to our local laboratory for a few booster shots and then we were to return in four weeks and get new immunoglobulin levels read again.

I also searched for prescription foot orthotics. We had to travel a half hour away to a specialty store for the insert molding appointment, then follow up for the fitting a few weeks later. Joshua also had his annual endocrinology appointment up in Weymouth that time of year. He had developed reactive hypothyroidism from the lithium prescription. I also had to find a geneticist as well as a pediatric cardiologist to make sure there were no heart abnormalities. (The echocardiogram came back crystal clear.) Of course we were required to see Dr. Jones every few months. I was also told I should find a pediatric ophthalmologist down on the Cape who could look behind Joshua's retina to determine potential genetic disorders.

Did I mention the urologist too? This was at Joshua's request, as he was ten-years-old and still experiencing difficulty with nighttime bedwetting. He longed to have a slumber party or sleepover without worrying about being embarrassed by an accident. These specialists, paired with his after school therapeutic program and two other children very involved in sports, left me haggard.

When I finally cried out for help, our case manger from DMH suggested I request a medical case manager through my insurance company Blue Cross Blue Shield. I submitted the paperwork, and the case manager assigned was truly helpful with finding me available specialists. Yet the onus was still on me to organize these appointments all in different areas of the state.

There was one more idea I could try—the Complex Care Program up at Children's Hospital. The program takes medically complicated children and provides a physician to oversee treatment and coordinate necessary appointments. Although this sounded like a Godsend, I had to get Joshua's pediatrician on board. A few weeks and phone calls later, I received his blessing to pursue this program. Once I pleaded Joshua's case with Complex Care, I awaited their response. Three weeks later I was finally in!

Happy Feet

Joshua was advised to stop all antibiotics one week prior to the first surgery so that there was a line of defense the physicians would have in the event he acquired an infection. Obediently I stopped the antibiotics that week, but I did not tell the school. After three days of no antibiotics, the school scheduled a progress review and brought up their concerns. Apparently, Joshua had substantially regressed during that week. They were horrified to see his reading fluency decrease by nearly twenty words per minute. Joshua could no longer compute basic math facts. His attention declined, his fine motor skills regressed, and his tics were returning. Joshua lost all sense of his body awareness in space; he was falling out of chairs and stumbling through the classroom.

Even I had to admit that he could not get through simple homework assignments and that he seemed more frustrated and irritable. They were very concerned. I quickly apologized for not disclosing sooner that Joshua was off the antibiotics that week. We were all amazed at the massive impact they continued to have on his functioning and quality of life! Often when something improves quickly, you get used to it and do not appreciate its positive changes after awhile. We were simply used to Joshua's current level of functioning. This was a tough couple of weeks on Joshua, but very valuable in reminding us how much the antibiotics continued to help him enjoy his life with fewer struggles.

The morning of the first surgery finally arrived. Grammy and I escorted Joshua up to Children's at the early hour of four in the morning. Dr. Mahan released the tendons, muscles, and fascia around the ankle, sides, and top of the foot to expedite the required drop of his high arch in preparation of the second surgery two weeks later. After an extensive four hour wait, I was allowed to sit beside him while he awoke from anesthesia. He looked so peaceful while he slept. I prayed in a hushed voice that Joshua would remain in peaceful slumber just a little bit longer. Finally, Joshua awoke quite groggy and thirsty. The first thing he saw was me, and the second thing was his special teddy bear, Pal, sleeping beside him with a matching rainbow cast.

"Hi buddy, how do you feel?"

"Rrrhhmm," Josh whimpered.

"Mommy is here. You will be okay. I won't leave you."

"But mommy, where is my foot? It hurts yet I can't feel it."

"That's just the anesthetic keeping it numb right now."

"Don't leave me, Mommy."

"Never."

In recovery they warned Joshua not to drink too much juice, because he had not eaten in over twenty-four hours. But with parched lips and sunken eyes, the nurses eventually watched him successfully drink a juice box. Later that afternoon, Joshua was released from post operative care with another juice box on his lap. As we waited in the lobby for my car to be delivered from valet parking, Joshua waited in his wheelchair. As his head bobbed side to side in and out of sleep, he slowly inhaled that second juice box. Anesthesia still running through his veins, I hauled him out of the wheel chair and he laid his head on my lap, stretching across the cushioned couch while we waited. Thank God it was a vinyl couch.

I gently petted Joshua's hair and sang soothing songs when he abruptly sat up, made a wretched noise, and started vomiting everywhere. It was all over the cushions, the floor, and especially him! The rancid smell, Joshua's hanging head, and my crazed eyes touched the most compassionate hearts. About five parents all ran to assist me. While one mother fetched paper towels, another watched Joshua while I ran into the gift shop and picked out a "Life is Good" set of pajamas. Ironic. Another mother held up a blanket so I could maintain some sense of privacy for Joshua while changing his clothes in the middle of the lobby traffic. There was never a dull moment!

I could not fathom that Dr. Mahan's prediction that Joshua would be weight bearing on his walking cane within three days, but he did! He only missed one day of school; when he returned, he felt like a superstar because every child wanted to sign that rainbow cast. My heart swelled with cheerfulness when I witnessed Joshua's resiliency. The first two weeks were a pleasure cruise compared to the second surgery and its recovery.

The second procedure was scheduled two weeks later. Dr. Manning performed an osteotomy (bone removal) from the large tarsal bone on the inside of the foot, manipulated it, and then replaced it with a human cadaver bone graft. She also performed tendon transfers to the first three toe tendons so that they would no longer curl under. Grammy came with me for moral support. It was a very long day; we arrived at six in the morning to begin the lengthy registration process which included a complete physical. The surgery began at ten. The procedure was not complete until three that afternoon, Joshua was in recovery until five that evening, and I did not leave his hospital room until seven. God bless Dave for volunteering to spend the night at the hospital on their wretched sleeping chair.

There are few other types of pain which can compare to deep bone pain from foot surgery. Joshua awoke on morphine and dilaudid. He remained in the hospital until the following afternoon, and then he was discharged in a wheelchair. I purchased a portable toilet, and a seal proof bag to protect his cast when in the shower. Dave prepared the house by making space for medical equipment in his bedroom and setting up a long ramp in our garage. However, nothing could have prepared us for the inconvenience of trudging him and that chair through the heavy, wet snow. The snow was excessive that winter, and the dirty, black snow was all over everything. It stuck to the wheels; it dripped all over our hardwood floors. I heaved and pushed. We tried to make the best of it though as we pushed him kamikaze-style down the icy driveway slope.

The first week our only priority was pain management. I would cringe watching his torment. We gave him my grandfather's antique copper bell to ring whenever he needed anything. We took turns at night sleeping on the couch so we could administer the medication every four hours. Joshua has always been the best patient I knew. I'll never forget the first sponge bath I gave him about four days post surgery. Lying on his bedroom floor I attempted to wash him gently while his body trembled and face wrinkled in agony. Silent tears rolled down his cheeks while his body lay limp on the ground. Yet he never complained...never. Oh how I wished I could bottle up for myself his courage and humility.

The two surgeries combined resulted in Joshua being casted and wheelchair bound for a total of eight weeks. During that time, I developed a newfound respect for families who need to make their homes wheelchair accessible as well as transport this equipment. I could barely lift the wheelchair! Every time I hauled it in and out of the car I would break a sweat. It was physically taxing on Joshua as well. After a few weeks, he got sick of the wheelchair, and left to his own devices, he just scooted everywhere through the house on his bum.

After the second cast was removed, the stark difference between the two feet was inconceivable. His right foot was three sizes longer than the left! The arch had dropped significantly, and his toes were straight! After six more weeks of physical therapy, Joshua preferred his right foot. The entire process lasted about four months.

After purging the house of ramps and medical equipment, I informed Dr. Mahan I wanted to wait to repeat this process on his left foot until the end of the summer. Joshua missed out on so many sports and activities during the winter and spring. This was the least I could do. I wanted to see my guy running on the beach and jumping into the deep end at Grammy's pool! I dreamed of him having fun camping and taking a much deserved break.

The left foot was scheduled for August, and before the surgery, we returned to Dr. Mahan to overview the pending procedure as well as get a final comparison of the two feet side-by-side. It was easy to get caught up in the excitement that day as Dr. Mahan eagerly brought in medical students and colleagues to show them the miraculous transformation of Joshua's right foot. Everybody gushed and congratulated the doctor; I felt like I just had a baby or won the lottery! Dr. Mahan asked if I would consider allowing Joshua's feet to be professionally photographed and videographed for the greater good of science and medicine. We laughed as we teased Joshua about his soon-to-be famous feet. There felt like no greater privilege. Joshua was elated, bouncing on cloud nine as we went down to the studio. The funniest part of the entire thing was that every time the photographer would snap a picture of Joshua's feet, he would pose a cheesy smile! He really thought fame and fortune were around the corner. I giggled to myself and soaked in this moment. He'd earned it! And I felt joy.

After a full recovery Joshua joined the town basketball team for the first time. He enjoyed being an integral player. We delighted seeing him pursue an active role on defense with and develop great rebound skills. He seemed larger than life on the basketball court and loved the competition. I suppose I was a little nervous having Joshua play sports; his feet were still tender with scars and I didn't know if he could handle the pressure. During one particularly intense game I crossed the line… unintentionally.

The fourth quarter was closing in and the big lead that Joshua's team originally had was dwindling. I could see the concern shade over Joshua's face. His eyes darted from the clock to the ball to the clock to the players. With only one minute left in the game, I saw a fierce determination sweep over Joshua's expression. As an opposing player caught the ball, Joshua's piercing look may have screamed "That ball will be mine!" Quickly Joshua jumped behind the player and wrapped his arms around the boy's shoulders and neck. He started tugging and pulling up on the ball from behind as if his life depended on it. Joshua was virtually at risk of choking the other player during the frenzy.

Suddenly, out of nowhere, a sound emerged and exploded throughout the gym. Moments later I realized with horror that sound was from deep within…me! It was my own voice. I prolonged each word as it escaped my lips in a howl. "Joshy… No! Let it go!" I bellowed. Then there was an uncomfortable silence as forty sets of parents poked their heads out from the edge of the sidelines to stare at me. Immediately Joshua dropped the ball and walked over to where I stood. He dramatically threw his hands out to his sides and yelled "What mom?" With all eyes on me, I timidly replied, "Never mind, go back and play honey" with a smile on my face. *Boy am I going to get it bad tonight!* I thought. Joshua was extremely mad at me for embarrassing him and I felt awful. But to my own defense, I could not stop the scream that emerged. Call it a mother's instinct. But I will always know I did the right thing that day because I saw the flash in his eyes—I saw his eyes go green—when nobody else did. But I still haven't lived the incident down. In the end, Joshua finished a successful basketball season, making it all the way to the final championship game!

SETBACKS

Joshua was prescribed eight pills in the morning and ten pills at night for mood stabilization, Lyme disease antibiotics, and to control the unwanted side effects of these drugs. It was just way too many pills. Since Joshua's feet were healing, I tentatively tried to decrease his medication with my psychiatrist's blessing. My biggest concern was the lithium. While I knew lithium was a potent defense for mood dysregulation, I was concerned about Joshua's kidneys. Urological studies indicated that his kidneys were working overtime, and that he was producing three times the normal amount of urine. To combat this side effect, he took six additional pills each evening. The lithium also caused hypothyroidism, resulting in one more extra pill in the mornings. I theorized that if we could get him slowly off the lithium, that would drastically reduce the amount of medicine he needed.

The first few weeks after we reduced the Lithium everything seemed status quo. But within one month the depression, tears, and agitation became Joshua's constant companion. Whenever Joshua was sent to his room I could hear him talking to himself in self deprecating ways with comments such as, "I hate myself! I wish I would die! I'm stupid! Nobody loves me!" Joshua slipped quickly in and out of this fragile emotional state.

Finally, after a horrid fight with Caleb, I sat him down for a heart to heart chat. With my arms wrapped tightly around his shaking shoulders I asked, "Joshua, are you happy?"

"No, Mama."

"Joshua, do you want to increase your medicine so you feel better?"

"Mama, I don't want more medicine, and I don't want to feel this way either."

"Oh sweet boy," I said, "We've tried, but it looks like you just can't have it both ways. You have to pick."

With a big gulp and a heavy sigh, Joshua straightened his posture and claimed, "Then I choose to feel happy. Give me the medicine."

I prodded further and asked, "Josh, what else do you need?"

He replied, "I think I need help Mama, but I'm afraid to leave you." My heart crumbled. I reassured him it was okay to ask for help and that it was a sign of his maturity. I explained how I would call Mobile Crisis and they could come out and give us some options that could help him. With resignation, Josh sobbed as he embraced his snuggle bug dog Cinamin.

Luckily I had just finished crafting a Crisis Plan, which I was able to put into effect. The required Alexa to call Grammy and Grampy and ask for their assistance, and it had all crucial contacts easily accessible. Dave rushed home from work while we waited for Mobile Crisis to arrive. Joshua freely talked to the social workers about his suicidal ideation and anxiety over his relationship with his father. Josh admitted that he also hurt himself when he's alone in his bedroom by punching and slapping his body. He claimed he did that to try to make the pain go away. *Oh sweetness, let me ease your pain*, I thought.

We finally agreed on a plan that would provide Joshua with the best treatment options, but it meant that I had to sleep on a small cot with him at the Crisis Center while we waited for a bed to open at Franciscan Hospital. I knew the arrangement was a merciful gesture that kept us from sleeping on gurneys in the hospital's emergency room hallway, but I felt so alone.

When we told him it was time to leave, gut wrenching sobs spewed like a volcanic eruption. Joshua's loud, crackling wails were filled with fiery pain. I could not hold it in any longer;

I broke down. *How can I cry like this in front of my own child?* I chastised myself. I rushed out of the room and started to pack his clothes between sobs and Kleenex wipes. As we left the house Josh started saying farewell to everything in his sight. "Farewell house, farewell mailbox. Farewell tree, farewell family. Farewell lights, farewell kitties." Then he started crying out to God, "Please help me God, please!" I couldn't take any more of this melodramatic farewell; I cursed myself for not being strong enough. I felt searing, blistering pain ripping through my core as I helplessly watched Joshua suffer. I simply could not bear to listen to his wailing any longer. *I've spent my whole life running away from pain! God, why are you throwing it in my face again?* I desperately prayed. I tried to turn on music, but he cried out over the top of that. The ten minute car ride felt like a long nightmare.

As we settled into our tiny room Joshua was able to calm down and he finally slept. On the other hand, I curled into a ball on a small freezing cot. I tried to remind myself whenever my anxiety set in that God had plans for Joshua and that he is a GIFT from God. His angels were watching over us. I was determined to embrace the sleeplessness if it meant peace for my son.

I knew in my heart once Joshua was safe and secure in the hospital that a peace would fall upon us. By this point we had prayer warriors calling out to God's angels and we were covered in that reassurance. Sure enough, as Dave and I said goodbye there were no tears this time. Joshua felt safe and loved. We finally arrived back at home by ten at night; the entire process lasted thirty hours.

During this hospitalization Joshua's medication was not adjusted. Instead, the focus centered on our family dynamics and Joshua's increased anxiety about meeting his father's expectations. Consequently, Dave agreed to pursue counseling and spend more time bonding with Joshua. Within six days Joshua's depression had lifted and he was excited to come home for a new beginning. The hospitalization provided Joshua with a gift of an insurance-paid holiday!

LIFE GOES ON

The family was ready to celebrate Joshua's road to recovery. We decided to take a vacation over spring break on a western Caribbean cruise to the lush, island of Cozumel. Cozumel is known for its picturesque landscapes, rolling waves, and abundance of tropic fish. Josh could not have been more thrilled. He was such a trooper, walking (and running) around in his walking cast after foot surgery. Joshua was able to stay out late at night participating in the kids' activities and even opted to stay behind with his peers while we snorkeled around the reefs of Cozumel! He was growing up so fast.

By May Joshua was out of the walking cast. Now the foot that was operated on was three sizes bigger than the other! The only solution was to purchase a pair of Keen sandals which supported his feet from every angle. Joshua also endured two months of rigorous physical therapy; he worked so hard!

As Joshua continued to improve physically and emotionally, I was uncertain whether he should attend summer school. After two surgeries and six months in and out of the wheelchair, he earned lazy beach days, long dips in his grandmother's pool, a camping adventure, sleepy mornings, play dates, and vacation bible school. Ultimately this became the first summer in which I did not send him.

Joshua's fifth grade year had been full of social growth. My heart soared when he asked a new friend to attend Caleb's birthday roller racer party. I was impressed at Joshua's choice for a friend—someone who was quite, kind, polite—much like himself! Joshua was beaming at the birthday party. This year he made more friends because he spent more time in the regular classroom. His lunches were filled with new friends, stories, and laughter. I was thrilled beyond belief. Joshua learned how to be a better friend to his peers and siblings. Although Joshua's relationship with Caleb still shows the strain of two competitive brothers, his relationship with Alexa has improved tremendously. I catch them giggling, watching movies, and playing sports more often.

Nevertheless, since Joshua's emotional needs lessened, DMH phased out their services. I reluctantly said goodbye to our case manager of the past six years Arvella Hagan. She kindly referred us to Baystate Services covered by Joshua's secondary insurance Mass Health. Through Baystate we participated in family therapy for a few months. I also secured a mentor for Joshua that I could trust. James Delano, an amazing, godly, young man from our church offered to be a role model and friend to Joshua. They consistently spend time together every Sunday afternoon. Joshua delights in this friendship.

Joshua's trials and tribulations are not over; he will inevitably struggle with some degree of disability or illness his entire life. But it will be a blessed life. He will gain spiritual wisdom and be able to teach others about his own journey.

A Gentle Soul

Watching Joshua triumph over many obstacles and witnessing the happiness he creates for himself is truly inspiring. The contentedness that Joshua exudes no matter what life brings reminds me of the character Forrest Gump. Like Forrest, Joshua may always be simple-minded yet he will continue to live a blessed, amazing life full of love and warmth. He has and will continue to make a difference in this world. He already has motivated and inspired many others.

Being the most popular, best looking, or most successful person means nothing to Joshua. When I see peace and contentment amidst the adversity which spills out of Joshua's heart, I know that worldly success and intelligence just don't matter. These things are not as important as Joshua's generosity, compassion, resilience, and faith.

Joshua teaches me mercy. The Lord's mercy reigns down constantly, yet many choose to stifle an extension of that mercy onto others. Many people who have not struggled have minimal empathy or patience for those who do. The Lord has pruned me through Joshua's circumstances and I pray he will continue to do so throughout the years. The winding road God has placed me and Joshua upon has blessed me with empathy, mercy, and compassion for suffering families and children.

Joshua encompasses simplicity. He is simply simple! He does not talk much of yesterday (unless it's Disney World or Six Flags), and the future is too ethereal for him to grasp. He acknowledges what's in front of him. And oh, how he prays. It is not always graceful or eloquent, but he is my one child who wears his heart on his sleeve. He never hesitates to lead grace at dinner or ask God to bring Daddy home safely from work every day.

Most Sunday's at the morning worship you can find Joshua excitedly raising his hand to share a celebration with the congregation, even if it is only, "My birthday is six months away!" The people chuckle, and Joshua beams. He adores everybody at church and knows he is safe there.

Joshua teaches me gentleness. He only wants to love and be loved. His gentle spirit longs to have a family someday—to find a wife he can love, with children and animals to care for and raise. *How many eleven-year-olds want this?* I wonder. This past year, after one of our many trips to Children's Hospital, Joshy looked around at the combination of doctors, nurses, and volunteers in the lobby while we waited for our car. He gently tugged my arm and said, "Mommy, when I grow up, if I can't work at Disney World, I want to work at Children's so I can help other children like me."

Joshua is the most generous person I know. When he gets birthday money, he offers to spend it on the *family!* There are no requests for video games or toys Instead, Joshua takes his siblings to the movies and the arcade with his allowance. Joshua's primary purpose is to show his love and appreciation to his family at all costs.

Joshua is also generous with his time and abilities. Despite having weak and achy hands, he is always beside me willing to rub my shoulders each night. He is in tune to my aches and pains and whether I'm tired, angry, happy, or sad. His empathy and attentiveness to other's needs is remarkable.

HEALING

Joshua's healing progresses and evolves every day. Joshua and I returned to New Haven to visit Dr. Jones during late summer 2011. He had been on antibiotics for eighteen months by that time. After Dr. Jones completed a thorough examination, Joshua hurried himself out to the lobby where the video games awaited.

"Jamie, I am so impressed with Joshua. Every time he visits his eyes look more engaged and alert. But this time he eyes are so bright and sparkly!?

"Really? Are you sure? I don't think I noticed that on my own."

"I see peace and joy in his eyes that once did not exist."

"Now you're pulling my leg, Dr. Jones. You truly see that?"

"I do! Nurse! Go look at Joshua's eyes in the lobby and tell me what you see."

"They're sure sparkly Dr. Jones!"

"Jamie, how are his tics?" I thought for a moment.

"Actually, I nearly forgot that was a monumental concern long ago. They're gone!"

"What about his mood?"

"He continues to take mood stabilizers, but since he started antibiotics, he has not required medication changes or struggled with mood swings! Now that I think about it, Joshua has made it through the summer without difficulty!"

Dr. Jones probed further.

"Is there anything else that has greatly improved?"

"Now that you mention it, his social skills and adherence to authority are a little better. A huge success for Josh this summer was that he was able to attend the town's Camp Clark Summer

Program *independently* without incident! He has been able to navigate social relationships and follow routines and rules."

Together we marveled at Joshua's victories throughout his amazing uphill battle. I asked Dr. Jones if he thought that the exposure to the Lyme has caused all of Joshua's symptoms.

"The exposure could have either *caused* everything, or it could have exacerbated predisposed tendencies that may have already been in Joshua's genetic makeup. We do have the genetic results indicating he carries the CMT 1A gene. There was a good chance this condition would not be severe at this early age, but because of Lyme exposure, Joshua's CMT 1A symptoms were released throughout his neuromuscular system with a vengeance."

"Well, I do agree with that. My genetic testing was returned this week, and it confirmed I have CMT 1A as well. But I do not have severe symptoms at twice his age, nor have I been exposed to Lyme disease."

"Exactly!"

I disclosed to Dr. Jones that in my heart of hearts, I *knew* that except for the CMT 1A, all of Joshua's symptoms were a manifestation of Lyme exposure. I fought with doctors, psychiatrists, insurance companies, the public schools, and even my family for over a decade and today I am blessed with healing, peace, and understanding.

Of these things I am certain: Joshua's future will be bright, colorful, and full of joy that only God can bestow. My life will forever be intertwined with Joshua and I have peace with this. Our road ahead may have twists and turns, but God has proven to me over and over again he will never leave our side. There is blessed assurance in knowing that together Joshua and I will have eternity in God's kingdom.

Through Joshua I have learned that healing is so much more than one miraculous moment when disease is obliterated. God provides healing in so many other creative ways; he provides beautiful and wondrous methods beyond my wildest imagination.

The Lord heals through nature, music, and art. He heals through the creative supports he places in my life. He heals through the expertise of physician's minds and hands. He heals through research and psychiatrists. He heals through creativity, dreams, and tears.

Sometimes the Lord does not heal in a lightning bolt moment, but instead it happens gradually over time. Sometimes the healing is only in one specific area, for the rest is yet to come. Sometimes smaller versions of healing give me enough strength to carry on. Even more amazing, sometimes God heals in areas I do not ask for while leaving my original plea alone. God always knows what is best for me and he will never forsake me.

I experience emotional and spiritual healing with the passing time and concerted effort every day. After years of searching, I experienced massive relief when I was finally able to confirm Joshua's diagnoses. The obsession and scrutiny over the cause of what made Joshua "Joshua" were put to rest. This insight has filled me with acceptance and gratitude for the trials I have endured as his mother. The gift of Joshua's life will unequivocally continue to bring glory to God's name.

REFERENCES

Allen C. Steere. (2001). Lyme Disease. *The New England Journal of Medicine, 345:* 115-25. American Psychiatric Association. (2000). *Diagnostic and statistical manual of mental disorders* (4th ed., text rev.). Washington, DC: Author.

Bob Clark. (Director), & Jean Shepherd. (Writer). (1983). *A Christmas Story* [Motion picture]. (Available from MGM)

B. James, H. Lindsey. (2005). Jesus Take the Wheel [Recorded by Carrie Underwood]. On *Some Hearts* [CD]. Nashville, TN: Arista.

B. Webb-Mitchell. (1993). *God Plays Piano Too: The Spiritual Lives of Disabled Children*. New York: Crossroad Publishing Company.

Barry Adams (1999-2011). In Father Heart Communications (Ed.), *The Father's Love Letter*. Retrieved from http://fathersloveletter.com

Carol Stock Kranowitz, M. A. (1998). *The Out of Sync Child : Recognizing & Coping with Sensory Processing Disorder*. New York: Penguin Press.

Centers for Disease Control, & Prevention. (2011, May). Reported Lyme Disease Cases by State, 1999–2009. In *Lyme Disease* (Statistics). Retrieved from http://www.cdc.gov/lyme/stats/chartstables/reportedcases_statelocality.html

Charcot-Marie-Tooth Disease. (2011, August 20). Retrieved from http://en.wikipedia.org/wiki/Charcot%E2%80%93Marie%E2%80%93Tooth_disease

Chuck Harget. (2003). When The Wind Blows [Recorded by Point of Grace]. On 24</I> [CD Disc 2]. Nashville, TN: Word Entertainment.

Dimitri Papolos M.D., & Janice Papolos. (2006). *The Bipolar Child: The Definitive & Reassuring Guide to Childhood's Most Misunderstood Disorder* (3rd ed.). New York: Broadway Books. (Original work published 1999)

Dr. Charles Ray Jones. (2011, April). In Dr. Charles Ray Jones (Ed.), *Lyme & Tick-Borne Diseases*. Retrieved from http://www.drjoneskids.org/

Dr. Henry Wright. (2005). *A More Excellent Way: Be In Health–Spiritual Roots of Disease & Pathways to Wholeness*. Thomaston, GA: Pleasant Valley Publications. (Original work published 1999)

J. Leventhal PhD, L. Shea PhD. (2008). Neuropsychological and Neuropsychiatric Features of Lyme and Other Tick Borne Diseases. In L. Shea PhD. J. Leventhal PhD (Ed.), *Seminar* (Neurological and Neuropsychiatric Features of Lyme and Other Tick Borne Dieseases). Baltimore: Chesapeake ADHD Center of Maryland.

Kevin Cooley. (2011, June). *Moon Light Affects*. Retrieved from http://home.hiwaay.net/~krcool/Astro/moon/moonring/

Lymesite.com. (2011, June). In WordPress.com (Ed.), *Lyme Handbook*. Retrieved from http://www.lymesite.com/Dr%20 Jones%20why%20give%20support.htm

Mark Shultz. (2000). He's My Son [Recorded by Mark Shultz]. On *Mark Shultz* [CD]. Nashville, TN: Word Entertainment.

Mary Ann McDonnell, A. P. R. N. (2008). Is Your Child Bipolar? The Definitive Resource on How to Identify, Treat, and Thrive with a Bipolar Child. New York: Bantam Dell.

Merriam Webster, Inc. (2011). Control. In *Merriam-Webster Dictionary*. Retrieved from http://www.merriam-webster. com

Molindone. (2011, August 19). Retrieved from http://www. en.wikipedia.org/moban/wiki

Newton-Wellesley Hospital. (2009). [Final Report for Joshua Bierut]. Unpublished department of Pathology and Laboratory Services.

Nicole C. Mullen. (2007). One Touch (Press) [Recorded by Nicole C. Mullen]. On *Sharecropper's Seed* [CD]. Nashville, TN: Word Entertainment.

Regents of the Univeristy of Michigan. (2011). In Univeristy of Michigan Health System (Ed.), *Your Child Development & Behavior Resources: A Guide to Information & Support for Parents*. Retrieved from http: www.med.umich.edu/yourchild/index.htm

Richard Kramer. (n.d.). In Abbey Press (Ed.), *God Danced The Day You Were Born*. Retrieved August 10, 2001, from Christian Book Distributors Web site: http://www.Christianbook.com

Scott P. Richert. (2011). In The New York Times Company (Ed.), *The Guardian Angel Prayer*. Retrieved from About. Com Web site: http://www.catholicism.about.com/od/prayers/qt/Guardian_Angel.htm

Serum Sickness. (2011, August 23). Retrieved from http://en.wikipedia.org/wiki/Serum_sickness

Forrest Gump (1994) Tom Hanks, directed by Robert Zemekis, written by Winston Groom & Eric Roth, Paramount Pictures Hollywood CA

Topomax. (2011, August 24). Retrieved from http://en.wikipedia.org/wiki/Topamax

William P. Young. (2007). *The Shack*. Newbury Park, CA: Windblown Media.us!